BEGINNER'S GUIDE TO PALEO

Jumpstart Your Journey with a 28-Day Meal Plan

Stephen William

TABLE OF CONTENTS

Section 1: Understanding Paleo   **01**

Section 2: Preparing for Your Paleo Journey   **08**

Section 3: The 28-Day Paleo Meal Plan   **15**

- Week 1   **17**
- WeeK1 reflection   **38**
- Week 2   **42**
- WK2 reflection   **63**
- Week 3   **67**
- WK3 reflection   **88**
- Week 4   **92**
- WK4 Reflection   **113**

Section 4: What Next   **125**

SECTION 1 : UNDERSTANDING PALEO

DINING LIKE A DINOSAUR IN THE 21ST CENTURY

What?

Imagine if a caveman time-traveled to today's world. After getting over the shock of electric lights and smartphones, he'd probably be baffled by our food. "What's this 'microwavable meal' thing?" he'd grunt. Enter the Paleo Diet, which aims to mimic the eating habits of our Paleolithic ancestors. It's a culinary throwback to the era of hunters and gatherers, minus the need to actually hunt or gather (thank goodness for supermarkets!).

In essence, the Paleo diet is about embracing foods that are as close to their natural state as possible. It's a diet that's high in proteins and healthy fats, and low in grains and processed foods. Think of it as the diet Mother Nature might recommend if she wrote diet books.

How?

So how do we go about this ancient way of eating without a time machine? It's simpler than it sounds, and no, you don't need to wear a loincloth or carry a club (though, feel free to do so if it adds to the experience).

First, let's tackle the shopping list. If a caveman couldn't eat it, neither can you. This means your grocery trips should feel like a safari through the produce section and the butcher's aisle. You're looking for foods that could be hunted, fished, picked, or gathered. That's your new food pyramid right there.

Cooking is where it gets even more interesting. Say goodbye to processed sauces and hello to herbs and spices. Your kitchen will transform into a place where whole, unprocessed ingredients come together in a symphony of flavors, much like a harmonious gathering around a Paleolithic campfire.

In the Paleo world, creativity is key. Without grains, dairy, and processed sugars, you'll become a culinary MacGyver, finding ingenious ways to make classic dishes with Paleo-approved ingredients. Cauliflower rice becomes your new best friend, and almond flour is the unsung hero of your baking adventures.

The Paleo diet isn't just about eating differently; it's a lifestyle change. It's about connecting with your food in a way that's lost in today's fast-paced world. You'll learn to appreciate the natural flavors of food, the joy of cooking from scratch, and the satisfaction of knowing you're eating what nature intended.

And the best part? You get to do all this with the convenience of modern amenities. No need to start a fire in your backyard (unless you're into that sort of thing). The Paleo diet marries the ancient with the modern, showing us that sometimes, looking back is the best way to move forward in our health and wellness journey.
Why?
Now, onto the 'why' – why would anyone choose to eat like a caveman in an era of drive-thrus and food delivery apps? It's not just a quirky trend or a chance to brag about your primal eating habits; there's solid reasoning behind this dietary time travel.

- Genetic Blueprint Matching: Our genetic makeup hasn't changed much since the Paleolithic era. The theory is that our bodies are best adapted to the foods our ancestors ate. Modern diets, full of processed foods and sugars, are a stark departure from this. By eating Paleo, you're essentially feeding your body the type of fuel it was originally designed to run on.
- Nutrient Density: Paleo foods are nutrient powerhouses. Lean meats, fish, fruits, and vegetables are packed with vitamins, minerals, antioxidants, and other essential nutrients. These foods provide more bang for your nutritional buck, without the empty calories and additives found in processed foods.
- Avoiding Modern Diet Pitfalls: Many chronic diseases today are linked to dietary choices. The Paleo diet cuts out the usual suspects – refined sugars, trans fats, and high-glycemic carbohydrates. This means potentially lowering the risk of heart disease, diabetes, and other lifestyle-related conditions.
- Digestive Health: Our forebears didn't have processed grains and dairy, and some argue our digestive systems are still catching up. The Paleo diet is often seen as more 'gut-friendly,' helping to reduce inflammation and support gut health.

- Simplicity and Purity: There's something appealing about a diet that emphasizes simple, whole foods. It's a return to the basics, a culinary simplification in an overly complex world. This approach can lead to not only physical health benefits but also a more mindful, intentional relationship with food.
- Energy and Vitality: Many who adopt a Paleo lifestyle report higher energy levels and greater overall vitality. This could be due to the elimination of sugar spikes and crashes caused by processed carbs, leading to more stable energy throughout the day.
- Sustainable Weight Management: Rather than focusing on calorie counting, Paleo promotes a balanced approach to eating that naturally leads to weight regulation. By eating nutrient-dense, satiating foods, you're less likely to overeat or succumb to cravings.

In essence, the 'why' of Paleo is about harmonizing our modern lives with the wisdom of our past. It's a nod to our ancestors, acknowledging that in terms of diet, they might have had it right all along. The Paleo diet is more than just a way of eating; it's a step towards aligning our lifestyle with our evolutionary heritage, fostering health and wellbeing in a way that's both old and new.

EMBRACING THE PAST, NAVIGATING THE PRESENT

Foods to Keep - The Primal Pantry Staples

Proteins (Meat, Fish, Eggs):

- The cornerstone of the Paleo diet, these foods are what our hunter ancestors thrived on. Protein is essential for building and repairing tissues, making enzymes and hormones, and maintaining muscle mass and bone health.
- Lean Meats: Opt for grass-fed and pasture-raised options where possible. These meats are higher in nutrients like conjugated linoleic acid (CLA) and omega-3 fatty acids, which are known for their anti-inflammatory properties.
- Fish: Particularly fatty fish like salmon, mackerel, and sardines, are not only excellent protein sources but also rich in omega-3 fatty acids, which are crucial for heart and brain health. Aim for wild-caught to avoid potential contaminants found in some farmed fish.

- Eggs: Regarded as one of nature's most perfect foods, eggs are a powerhouse of nutrition, containing high-quality protein, healthy fats, vitamins, and minerals. They're also one of the few food sources of vitamin D.

Vegetables:
The variety and versatility of vegetables make them a staple in the Paleo diet. They provide essential nutrients and fiber, aiding in digestion and overall health.
- Leafy Greens: Spinach, kale, swiss chard, and other greens are loaded with vitamins A, C, E, and K, and minerals like iron and calcium.
- Cruciferous Vegetables: Broccoli, cauliflower, and Brussels sprouts are high in fiber and packed with cancer-fighting compounds.
- Root Vegetables: Carrots, beets, and sweet potatoes are more than just starch; they're great sources of vitamins, particularly vitamin A in the form of beta-carotene.

Fruits:
While higher in sugar, fruits in moderation can be a part of a healthy Paleo diet, offering a wealth of nutrients and antioxidants.
- Berries: Blueberries, strawberries, raspberries, and blackberries are among the best choices due to their high antioxidant content and lower glycemic impact.
- Citrus Fruits: Oranges, lemons, and limes provide vitamin C and flavonoids, which can boost immune function and skin health.

Nuts and Seeds:
These are not just for snacking; they can be ground into flours, used to make dairy-free milks, or added to dishes for texture and nutrition.
- Almonds and Walnuts: Both are good for heart health, rich in omega-3 fatty acids, and can improve cholesterol levels.
- Flaxseeds and Chia Seeds: These seeds are high in fiber and omega-3 fats, beneficial for digestive health and reducing inflammation.

Healthy Fats:
Fats are essential for hormone production, brain health, and absorbing vitamins. They also provide a slow and steady form of energy.

- Avocados: High in monounsaturated fats, they're great for heart health and maintaining healthy cholesterol levels.
- Olive Oil: Rich in antioxidants and monounsaturated fats, it's beneficial for heart health and has anti-inflammatory properties.
- Coconut Oil: Unique in its composition of medium-chain triglycerides (MCTs), it's a quick source of energy and may help in burning fat.

Foods to Avoid - The Agricultural Additions
Grains (Wheat, Barley, Oats):
- Grains were introduced during the agricultural revolution, making them a relatively new addition to the human diet from an evolutionary perspective. Here's why they are avoided in the Paleo diet:
- Gluten and Lectins: Many grains, especially wheat, contain gluten, which can cause digestive issues, inflammation, and autoimmune responses in some individuals. Lectins, another type of protein found in grains, can also irritate the gut lining and lead to similar problems.
- Anti-nutrients: Grains contain anti-nutrients like phytic acid, which can bind to minerals in the gut and prevent their absorption, potentially leading to deficiencies.
- High Glycemic Index: Grains are high in carbohydrates and can cause spikes in blood sugar, leading to energy crashes and, over time, contributing to insulin resistance and type 2 diabetes.

Legumes (Beans, Peanuts):
- Despite their nutritional value, legumes are not part of the Paleo diet for several reasons:
- Phytic Acid: Like grains, legumes contain phytic acid, which can hinder the absorption of minerals such as iron, zinc, and calcium.
- Lectins: These proteins can damage the gut lining, leading to digestive distress and contributing to conditions like leaky gut syndrome.
- Complex Sugars: Legumes contain complex sugars that can be difficult to digest, causing bloating and gas for some people.

Dairy:
- Dairy is typically excluded from the Paleo diet, primarily due to concerns about lactose and casein:
- Lactose Intolerance: Many people lack the enzyme lactase, which is needed to digest lactose, the sugar found in milk. This can lead to digestive issues like bloating, gas, and diarrhea.
- Casein Sensitivity: Casein, a protein in dairy, can trigger inflammatory responses in some individuals, similar to gluten in grains.

- Processed Dairy Products: These often contain added sugars, preservatives, and artificial ingredients, which are not aligned with the Paleo philosophy of eating whole, unprocessed foods.

Processed Foods and Sugars:
- The modern diet is rife with processed foods, which are antithetical to the Paleo approach:
- Unhealthy Fats and Additives: Processed foods often contain unhealthy trans fats, artificial flavors, and preservatives, which can contribute to chronic diseases.
- Refined Sugars: High consumption of refined sugars can lead to weight gain, metabolic disorders, and an increased risk of conditions like diabetes and heart disease.

Certain Vegetable Oils:
- Some vegetable oils are avoided due to their processing methods and fatty acid composition:
- High in Omega-6 Fatty Acids: Oils like soybean, corn, and canola are high in omega-6 fatty acids. While these are essential fats, an imbalance in the omega-6 to omega-3 ratio can promote inflammation in the body.
- Processing Methods: These oils are often heavily processed, which can involve high heat and chemical treatments, potentially resulting in harmful compounds.

By avoiding these food groups, the 28-day Paleo meal plan aims to reduce inflammation, improve digestion, and align more closely with the dietary patterns of our Paleolithic ancestors, potentially leading to improved overall health and well-being.

Grey Area Foods - The Personal Tolerance Test

Some Dairy (Fermented or High-Fat):
- In the strict Paleo diet, dairy is generally excluded, but there's a grey area for fermented or high-fat dairy products:
- Fermented Dairy: Products like yogurt and kefir are valued for their probiotics, which can improve gut health. The fermentation process reduces the lactose content, making these products more digestible for some people.
- High-Fat Dairy: Butter, particularly from grass-fed cows, is high in nutrients like butyrate, a fatty acid that can support gut health and reduce inflammation. It's also a good source of fat-soluble vitamins A, D, E, and K2.

- Personal Tolerance: The inclusion of these items depends on individual tolerance. Some people may find they can enjoy these foods without any adverse effects, while others may experience digestive discomfort or inflammation.

Certain Legumes (Green Beans, Peas):

- While most legumes are excluded from the Paleo diet, certain varieties like green beans and peas are often considered more acceptable:
- Lower in Phytic Acid and Lectins: Green beans and peas are lower in phytic acid and lectins compared to other legumes, making them easier to digest and less likely to interfere with nutrient absorption.
- Nutrient Profile: They are a good source of vitamins, minerals, and fiber, and can be a valuable addition to a balanced Paleo diet in moderation.
- Digestibility: These legumes are generally better tolerated, especially when cooked properly, which can further reduce any anti-nutrient content.

Starchy Vegetables (Sweet Potatoes):

- Starchy vegetables, particularly sweet potatoes, occupy a grey area in the Paleo diet:
- Nutrient-Dense: Sweet potatoes are packed with vitamins A and C, potassium, and fiber. They are an excellent source of carbohydrates for those who need more energy, such as athletes or highly active individuals.
- Carbohydrate Tolerance: The inclusion of sweet potatoes in a Paleo diet often depends on individual carbohydrate tolerance and energy needs. For some, they can be a healthy part of the diet, while others might need to limit their intake.

Natural Sweeteners (Honey, Maple Syrup):

- Natural sweeteners like honey and maple syrup are not strictly Paleo but can be used in moderation:
- Less Processed: Unlike refined sugars, honey and maple syrup undergo minimal processing and contain some nutrients and antioxidants.
- Glycemic Impact: While they are a healthier alternative to refined sugar, they still impact blood sugar levels and should be used sparingly, especially for individuals with blood sugar regulation issues.
- Flavor and Use: These sweeteners can add flavor to Paleo dishes and treats, but their use should align with the overall goal of reducing sugar intake.

SECTION 2: PREPARING FOR YOUR PALEO JOURNEY

Embarking on a Paleo lifestyle is like venturing into uncharted territory of ancient dietary habits. It's not just about swapping out a few ingredients; it's a holistic change that encompasses your environment, mindset, and daily routines. This preparation phase is crucial for a smooth transition and enduring success in your 28-day Paleo journey.

"BY FAILING TO PREPARE, YOU ARE PREPARING TO FAIL"

THE 5 STEPS

1. Assessing Your Environment: Creating a Paleo-Friendly Space

Transforming your kitchen into a Paleo haven is the first critical step on this prehistoric culinary adventure. Here's how to ensure your environment is perfectly primed for your Paleo journey.

Audit Your Pantry and Fridge:
- Comprehensive Review: Begin by thoroughly examining your current food inventory. Delve into every nook and cranny of your pantry and fridge.
- Identify Non-Paleo Items: Be on the lookout for common non-Paleo culprits like processed snacks, cereals, grains (such as wheat, barley, oats), dairy products, legumes (beans, lentils, peanuts), and any foods with added sugars or preservatives.
- Educate Yourself: This is also an educational opportunity to learn about hidden non-Paleo ingredients in seemingly harmless products. This knowledge is crucial for making informed choices when shopping.

Remove Temptations:
- Clean Sweep: Remove all non-Paleo foods. This isn't just about decluttering; it's a symbolic gesture of committing to your new lifestyle.
- Mindful Disposal: Consider donating unopened, non-perishable items to a local food bank. It's a responsible way to clear out non-Paleo items and support your community.
- Family Involvement: If you live with others, discuss how to handle shared food spaces. Maybe designate certain shelves or areas as Paleo-only.

Restock with Paleo Alternatives:
- Paleo Staples: Fill your pantry with essentials like nuts (almonds, walnuts), seeds (chia, flaxseeds), healthy oils (olive, coconut), and a variety of herbs and spices for flavor.
- Fresh Produce Galore: Emphasize fresh, organic vegetables and fruits. Think leafy greens, broccoli, peppers, avocados, berries, and apples.
- Quality Proteins: Stock up on grass-fed meats, wild-caught fish, and free-range eggs. These are not only more nutrient-dense but also align with the ethical ethos of the Paleo diet.
- Smart Swaps: Find creative alternatives like almond flour for baking, coconut milk for dairy, and cauliflower rice for grains.

Organize for Accessibility:
- Strategic Placement: Arrange your kitchen so that Paleo foods are the easiest to access. Keep fruits and nuts within easy reach for healthy snacking.
- Simplify Meal Prep: Organize ingredients in a way that streamlines your cooking process. Group items you frequently use together to save time and hassle.

Create a Paleo Information Center:
- Resource Corner: Dedicate a section of your kitchen for Paleo resources. This could be a shelf with cookbooks, guides, and a binder of your favorite recipes.
- Progress Journal: Include a journal or a board to track your progress, jot down meal ideas, or note foods that particularly work well for you.
- Inspirational Touch: Consider adding some motivational quotes or images that resonate with your health goals. This can be a daily reminder of why you embarked on this Paleo journey.

2. Crafting a Mindful Eating Space

Creating a mindful eating space is about nurturing an environment that complements your Paleo journey. It's where the act of eating transcends mere consumption and becomes a holistic experience. Here's how to cultivate such a space:

Dedicated Eating Area:

- Selecting the Right Spot: Choose a place in your home specifically for eating. This could be a part of your dining room, a cozy corner, or even a spot on your balcony with a view. The key is consistency – eating at this spot regularly reinforces mindful eating habits.
- Design Elements: Consider the ambiance. Soft, natural lighting, comfortable seating, and even some greenery or soothing artwork can make this space more inviting. The goal is to create an oasis where eating is not just necessary, but an enjoyable event.

Minimize Distractions:

- Tech-Free Zone: Implement a rule of no electronic devices at the table. This means no TV, smartphones, or tablets. It's about disconnecting from the digital world to connect with your food and the experience of eating.
- Quiet Environment: If possible, reduce background noise. Soft, instrumental music or the sounds of nature can be calming alternatives, but the focus should be on creating a quiet space that allows for introspection and attentiveness to your meal.

Comfortable Setting:

- Ergonomic Seating: Choose chairs that are comfortable yet supportive. Being physically comfortable is crucial for a relaxed meal where you can focus on the act of eating without distraction.
- Table Setting: Set your table with care. Use plates and utensils that you love, and consider adding a simple centerpiece like a vase of flowers or a small plant. This attention to detail can make each meal feel special.

Mindful Eating Techniques:

- Being Present: Before starting your meal, take a moment to truly settle in. Take a few deep breaths to center yourself and transition from the rush of the day to the calm of mealtime.
- Engage Your Senses: As you eat, engage all your senses. Notice the colors, textures, and smells of your food. When you take a bite, pay attention to the flavors and how they change as you chew.

- Chew Slowly: Take your time with each bite. Chewing slowly not only aids in digestion but also allows you to fully experience the taste and texture of your food.
- Listening to Your Body: Tune into your body's hunger and fullness signals. Eating mindfully means stopping when you're comfortably full, not when your plate is clean.

By establishing and nurturing a mindful eating space, you're not just eating to nourish your body; you're also feeding your soul. This mindful approach to dining can enhance your overall experience with the Paleo diet, making it more than a dietary change — a transformative lifestyle shift.

3. Mental Readiness: Embracing the Paleo Lifestyle

Adopting the Paleo lifestyle is as much a mental endeavor as it is a physical one. It's about equipping your mind to embark on this transformative journey. Here's how to cultivate the mental readiness necessary for embracing and thriving in the Paleo lifestyle:

Growth Mindset:
- View Paleo as a Learning Experience: Embrace the Paleo diet as an exciting opportunity to learn more about nutrition, cooking, and your body's needs. Each challenge is a chance to grow and expand your understanding.
- Celebrate Small Victories: Every time you choose a healthy Paleo meal over processed food, view it as a victory. These small wins accumulate to form significant lifestyle changes.
- Flexibility and Adaptability: Be open to adapting the diet to your needs. Paleo is not a one-size-fits-all approach, so give yourself permission to adjust as you learn what works best for you.

Positive Self-Talk:

Mindful Awareness: Pay attention to your inner dialogue. Are your thoughts mostly critical or encouraging? Actively work to shift towards more positive and supportive self-talk.

- Affirmations: Use affirmations to reinforce your commitment and reframe challenges. Phrases like "I am making choices that benefit my health" or "I am capable of overcoming cravings" are powerful motivators.
- Overcome Setbacks with Compassion: If you slip up, instead of berating yourself, acknowledge the slip as a learning opportunity. Remind yourself that progress is not linear and that resilience is key.

Support System:

- Community Engagement: Connect with others who are also following a Paleo lifestyle, either in your local community or online. Share recipes, experiences, and tips to support each other.
- Family and Friends: Involve your family or friends in your Paleo journey. Even if they are not following the diet, they can still offer support and encouragement.
- Professional Support: Consider consulting with a nutritionist or dietitian who is familiar with Paleo. They can offer tailored advice and guidance to ensure you're meeting your nutritional needs.

Reflective Practice to Enhance Mental Readiness:

- Weekly Reflections: Use your weekly reflections as a tool to assess not just your physical progress but also your mental and emotional states. Are you feeling more confident in your food choices? Are you finding joy in the Paleo lifestyle?
- Adjust Your Approach: Based on your reflections, adjust your mindset and strategies as needed. If you find certain aspects particularly challenging, brainstorm ways to overcome these hurdles.
- Document Insights and Inspirations: Keep a record of positive experiences and realizations. This can serve as a source of motivation and a reminder of how far you've come when faced with challenges.
- By nurturing a growth mindset, engaging in positive self-talk, building a strong support system, and using reflection as a tool for continuous improvement, you'll be well-equipped to embrace the Paleo lifestyle fully. This mental readiness is key to making the Paleo journey a rewarding and sustainable one.

4. Reflections: Tracking Your Progress Weekly

As part of preparing for your Paleo journey, setting up a structured reflection process is key. This involves regularly taking stock of various aspects of your health and well-being to understand how your body is responding to the Paleo diet. Here's how to incorporate and utilize the reflection layout effectively:

Schedule Regular Reflections
- Weekly Check-ins: Dedicate a specific time each week for your reflection session. Treat this as an essential part of your Paleo journey, just as important as meal planning or grocery shopping.
- Consistency: By consistently reflecting at the same time each week, you create a habit that fosters mindfulness and self-awareness.

Use the Rating System
- Objective Measurement: Utilize the provided rating scale to objectively measure changes in various health aspects, such as digestive comfort, energy levels, and mood. This scale helps quantify your experiences, making it easier to track progress over time.
- Detailed Notes: Alongside the ratings, keep detailed notes on each category. For example, if you rate your energy levels high, note what meals or habits might have contributed to this.

Reflect on Patterns and Adjustments
- Identify Patterns: Look for patterns or trends over the weeks. Are there consistent improvements in certain areas? Are some aspects not improving as expected?
- Make Adjustments: Use these insights to make informed adjustments to your Paleo plan. For example, if you consistently note digestive discomfort, consider tweaking your fiber intake or meal composition.

Document and Review Progress
- Journaling: Keep a dedicated journal or digital document for your reflections. This not only helps in tracking your progress but also serves as a motivational tool to see how far you've come.
- Review and Celebrate: Regularly review your cumulative progress. Celebrate the milestones, no matter how small, and use them as motivation to continue your Paleo journey.

Integrating a structured reflection process into your preparation for the Paleo journey is crucial for its success. It allows you to make your Paleo experience truly personalized, adjusting as you learn more about how your body responds to different foods and lifestyle changes. This reflective practice is not just about monitoring progress; it's a tool for self-discovery and empowerment on your journey to better health.

5. Label Literacy: Understanding Paleo Labels

Developing label literacy is a key skill for anyone adopting a Paleo lifestyle. It involves understanding and interpreting food labels to make informed choices that align with Paleo principles. Here's how to enhance your label literacy:

Ingredients List:
- Prioritize Whole Foods: Look for products with simple, whole-food ingredients. The fewer the ingredients, the more likely it aligns with Paleo guidelines.
- Recognize Non-Paleo Ingredients: Develop an understanding of common non-Paleo ingredients and their aliases. This includes grains, sugars, artificial additives, and highly processed oils.
- Ingredient Order Matters: Ingredients are listed by quantity, from highest to lowest. A Paleo-friendly item will have its main ingredients as recognizable whole foods.

Natural vs. Processed:
- Understanding 'Natural': Be cautious of products labeled as 'natural.' This term is not strictly regulated and can be misleading. Products marketed as 'natural' can still contain processed sugars, grains, or artificial additives.
- Whole and Unprocessed Focus: The core of Paleo is about eating foods in their natural, unprocessed state. If a product seems overly processed or far removed from its natural form, it likely doesn't fit the Paleo criteria.

Allergen Information:
- Gluten and Dairy-Free Labels: These labels can be a good starting point as they often indicate the absence of two major non-Paleo groups - grains and dairy. However, gluten-free does not automatically mean grain-free.
- Cross-Check Ingredients: Even if a product is labeled gluten or dairy-free, check for other non-Paleo ingredients like soy, legumes, or added sugars.
- Beware of Cross-Contamination: If you are particularly sensitive to non-Paleo allergens (like gluten), pay attention to disclaimers about manufacturing processes to avoid cross-contamination.

Additional Tips:
- Familiarize with Paleo-Friendly Brands: Over time, you'll become familiar with brands that typically align with Paleo principles. This can simplify shopping, but always stay vigilant as product formulas can change.
- Use Technology: Consider using smartphone apps specifically designed for Paleo shopping. These can help you quickly determine if a product fits your diet.
- Stay Informed: Food labeling regulations and product formulations can change. Keeping yourself educated on these changes ensures your label literacy remains up-to-date.

SECTION 3: THE 28-DAY PALEO MEAL PLAN

Welcome to your 28-Day Paleo Meal Plan, a comprehensive guide designed to introduce you to a healthier, more natural way of eating. This plan is based on the principles of the Paleo diet, which emphasizes whole foods, lean proteins, healthy fats, and fresh vegetables and fruits. It's a journey back to the basics of human nutrition, focusing on food that our ancestors thrived on.

Each day of the plan includes recipes for breakfast, lunch, dinner, and a snack. These meals are crafted to not only be delicious but also to provide a balanced approach to a Paleo lifestyle. Whether you're new to Paleo or looking to revamp your eating habits, this plan is structured to support your health and wellness goals.

Meal Plan Structure:

- Recipes for One: Each recipe is designed for one person. However, if you're cooking for your partner, a guest, or your family, simply double or adjust the quantities accordingly.
- Daily Meals: Every day includes a fulfilling breakfast, a nutritious lunch, a satisfying dinner, and a healthy snack to keep your energy levels steady throughout the day.
- Hydration: We recommend drinking plenty of water throughout the day. Staying hydrated is key to supporting your health on this diet. You can also enjoy beverages like sparkling water, as well as coffee and tea in moderation.

Emphasis on Whole Foods:
The Paleo diet is all about whole, unprocessed foods. You'll find that the meals focus on quality proteins, an abundance of vegetables, and healthy fats. Fruits are enjoyed for their natural sweetness, and nuts and seeds are included for their nutrient density.

Flexibility and Adjustments:
Feel free to swap meals between days if you have a preference for certain recipes. The goal is to make this meal plan work for you and your lifestyle. Listen to your body and adjust portion sizes according to your hunger and fullness cues.

Enjoy the Journey:
Remember, this meal plan is more than just about following recipes; it's about exploring a new way of eating and enjoying the process. Notice how your body responds to these wholesome foods and embrace the changes in your health and well-being.

Let's embark on this Paleo journey together, discovering how a diet rich in natural foods can bring about transformative health benefits. Enjoy the flavors, the variety, and the simplicity of eating Paleo!

WEEK 1: EMBRACING THE BASICS

Welcome to Week 1 of your Paleo journey! This week is all about laying the groundwork and easing into the Paleo lifestyle. Focus on understanding the core principles of Paleo and start incorporating basic Paleo meals into your daily routine. Remember, this is the first step towards a healthier you, so take it one meal at a time.

BREAKFAST :

DAY 1

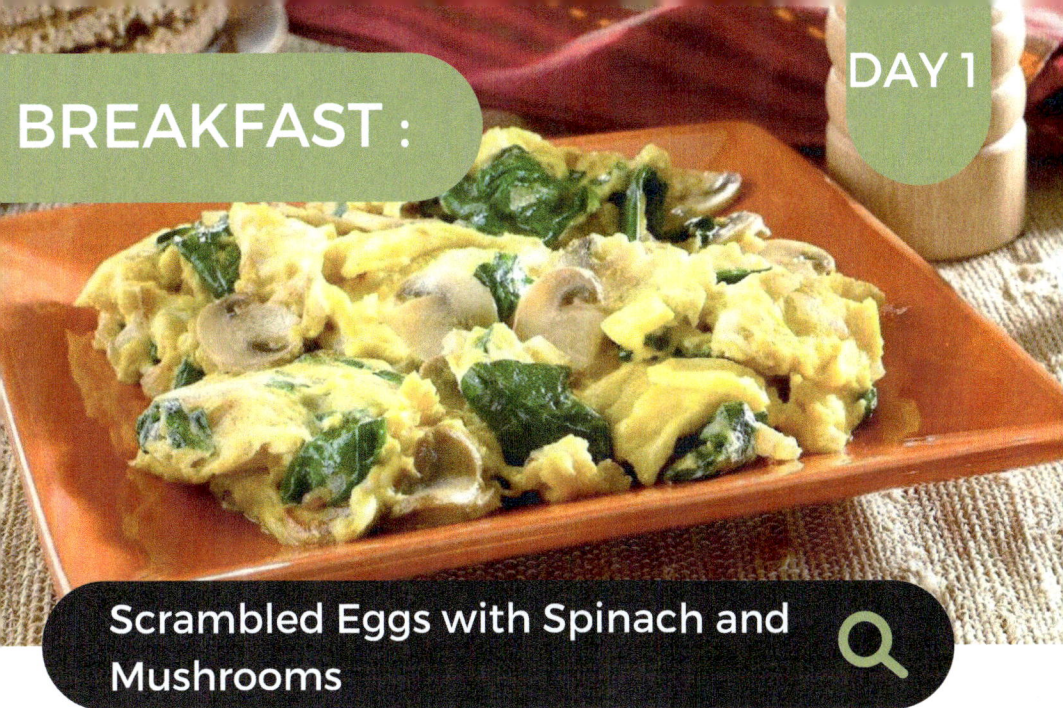

Scrambled Eggs with Spinach and Mushrooms

INGREDIENTS

- 2 large eggs
- 1 cup fresh spinach, chopped
- 1/2 cup mushrooms, sliced
- 1 tablespoon olive oil or coconut oil
- Salt and pepper, to taste

PROCEDURE

- Heat the oil in a skillet over medium heat.
- Add the mushrooms and sauté until they are soft, about 3-4 minutes.
- Add the spinach and cook until it wilts, about 1-2 minutes.
- Beat the eggs in a bowl and pour them into the skillet with the vegetables.
- Gently scramble the eggs with the vegetables until the eggs are fully cooked.
- Season with salt and pepper to taste.
- Serve hot.

PALEO DIET

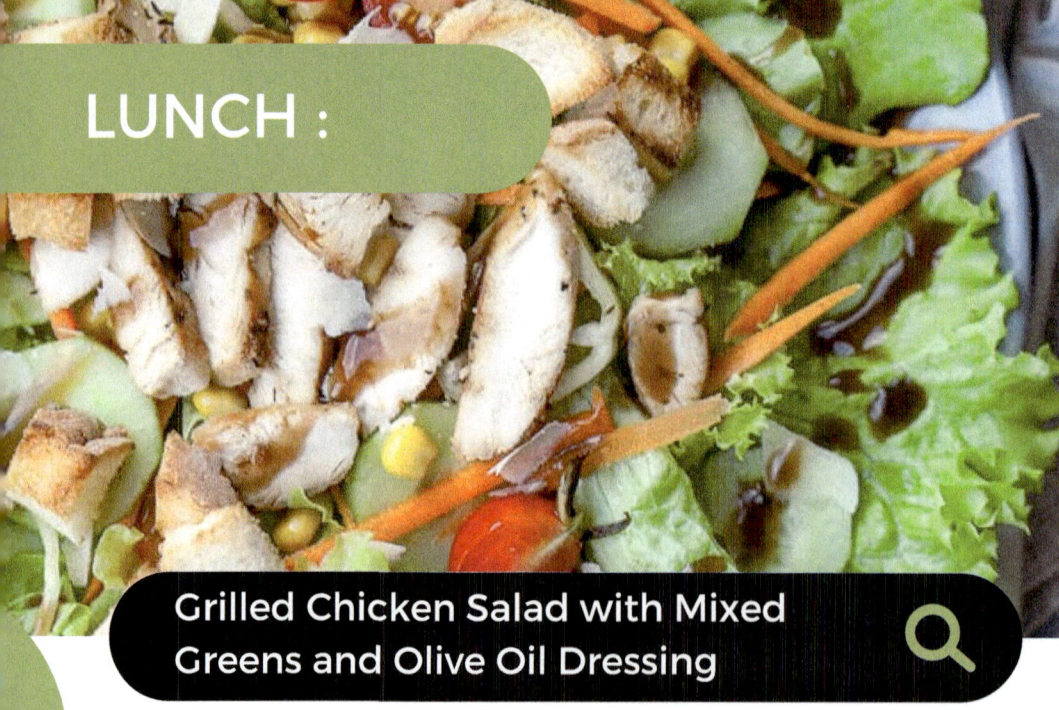

LUNCH :

Grilled Chicken Salad with Mixed Greens and Olive Oil Dressing

INGREDIENTS

- 1 small chicken breast
- 2 cups mixed greens (like lettuce, spinach, arugula)
- 1/2 cucumber, sliced
- 1/4 red onion, thinly sliced
- 2 tablespoons olive oil
- 1 tablespoon lemon juice
- Salt and pepper, to taste

PROCEDURE

- Season the chicken breast with salt and pepper.
- Grill the chicken over medium heat until it's fully cooked, about 6-7 minutes per side.
- Let the chicken rest for a few minutes, then slice it.
- In a large bowl, combine the mixed greens, cucumber, and red onion.
- In a small bowl, whisk together the olive oil and lemon juice, then season with salt and pepper.
- Toss the salad with the dressing.
- Top the salad with the sliced grilled chicken.
- Serve immediately.

PALEO DIET

DINNER :

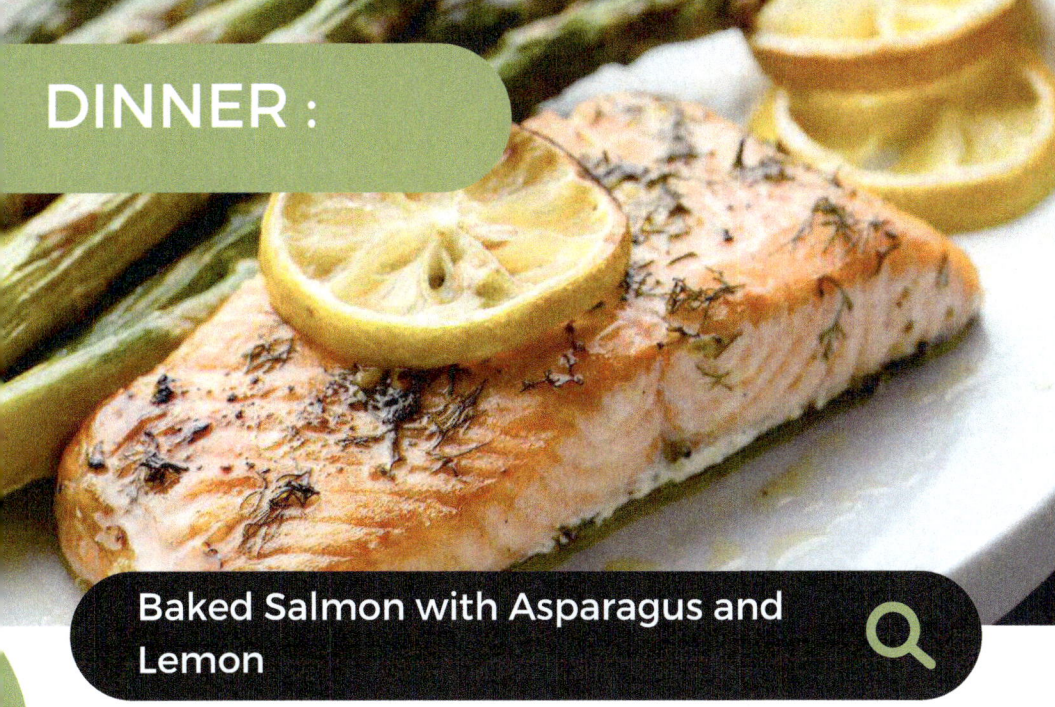

Baked Salmon with Asparagus and Lemon

INGREDIENTS

- 1 salmon fillet (about 6 oz)
- 1/2 bunch asparagus, ends trimmed
- 1 lemon, half sliced and half juiced
- 1 tablespoon olive oil
- Salt and pepper, to taste

PROCEDURE

- Preheat the oven to 400°F (200°C).
- Place the salmon fillet and asparagus on a baking sheet.
- Drizzle with olive oil and lemon juice.
- Season with salt and pepper.
- Place lemon slices on top of the salmon.
- Bake in the preheated oven for about 12-15 minutes, or until the salmon is cooked through and the asparagus is tender.
- Serve hot.

PALEO DIET

BREAKFAST :

DAY 2

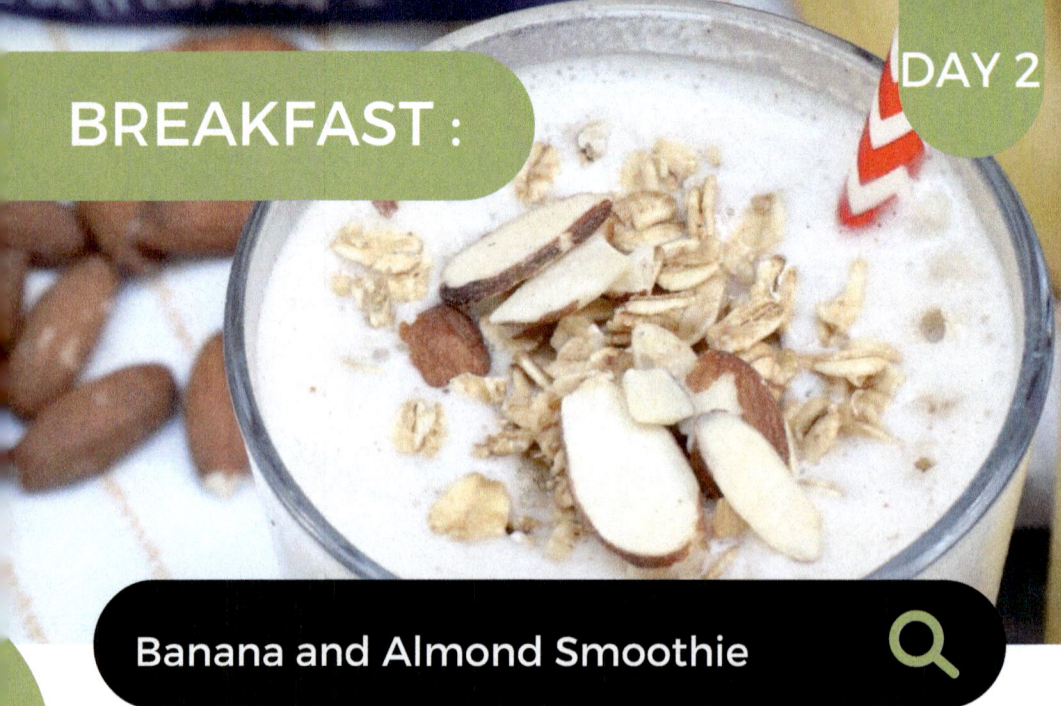

Banana and Almond Smoothie

INGREDIENTS

- 1 ripe banana
- 1/4 cup almond milk (unsweetened)
- 1 tablespoon almond butter
- A pinch of cinnamon
- Ice cubes (optional)

PROCEDURE

- Combine the banana, almond milk, almond butter, and cinnamon in a blender.
- Add ice cubes if desired for a colder smoothie.
- Blend until smooth and creamy.
- Serve immediately in a tall glass.

LUNCH :

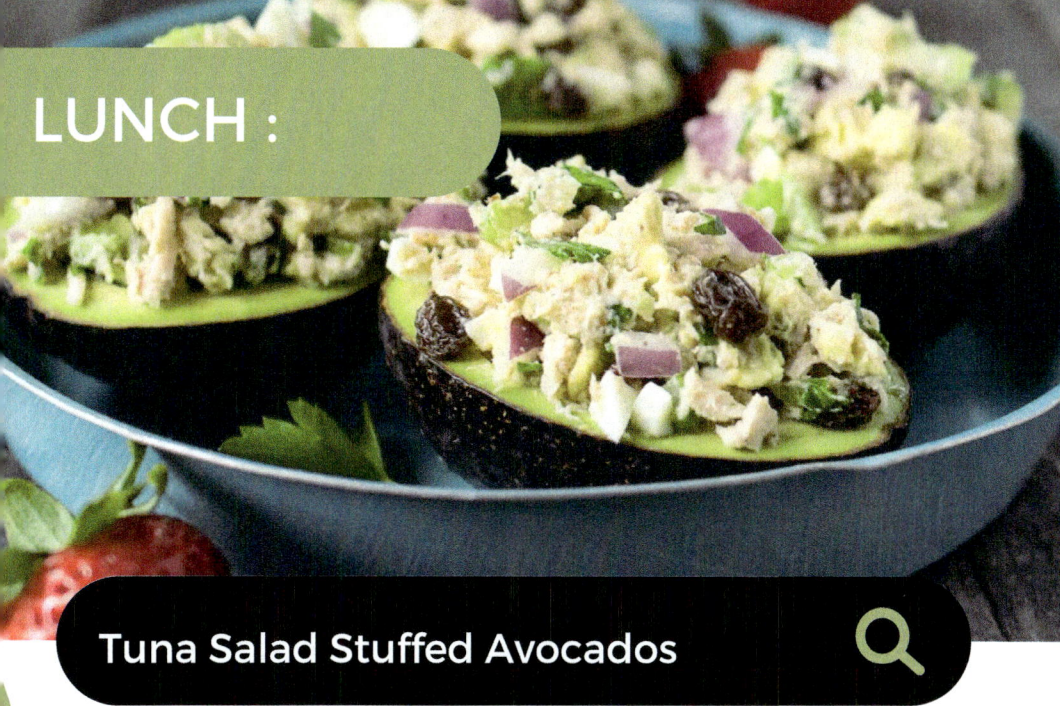

Tuna Salad Stuffed Avocados

INGREDIENTS

- 1 can of tuna in water, drained
- 1/2 ripe avocado
- 1 tablespoon diced red onion
- 1 tablespoon chopped celery
- 1 tablespoon olive oil
- 1 teaspoon lemon juice
- Salt and pepper, to taste

PROCEDURE

- In a bowl, mix the tuna, red onion, celery, olive oil, and lemon juice.
- Season the mixture with salt and pepper.
- Cut the avocado in half and remove the pit.
- Spoon the tuna mixture into the avocado halves.
- Serve immediately.

PALEO DIET

DINNER :

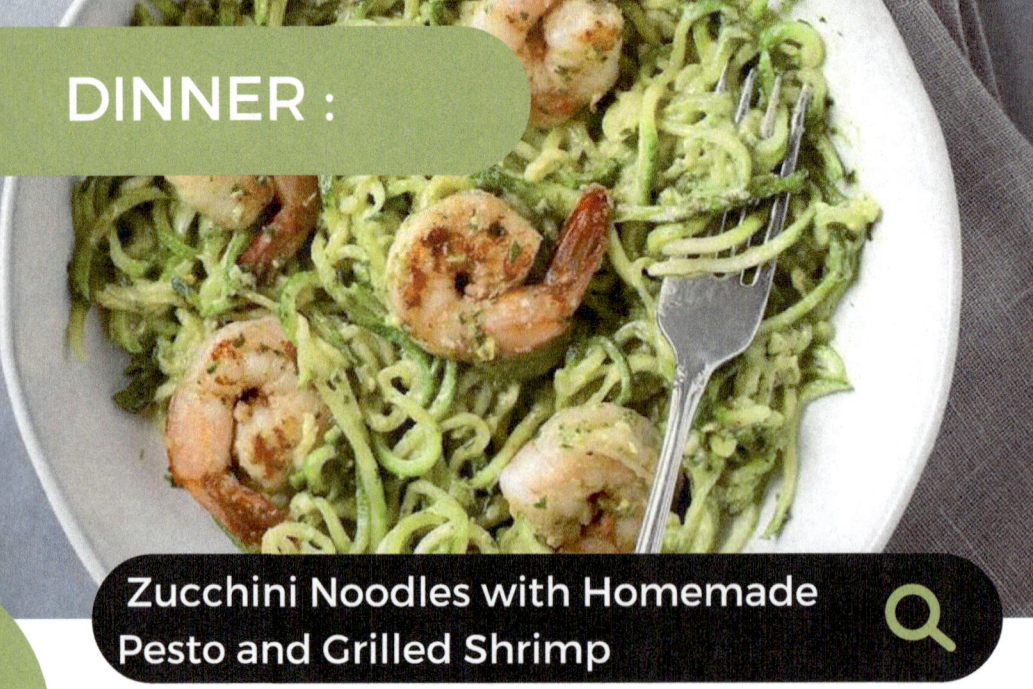

Zucchini Noodles with Homemade Pesto and Grilled Shrimp

INGREDIENTS

- 1 large zucchini
- 5-6 large shrimp, peeled and deveined
- 1/4 cup fresh basil leaves
- 1 tablespoon pine nuts or walnuts
- 1 garlic clove
- 2 tablespoons olive oil
- Salt and pepper, to taste

PROCEDURE

- Use a spiralizer to create zucchini noodles, or use a vegetable peeler for wider ribbons.
- For the pesto, blend basil, nuts, garlic, and 1 tablespoon of olive oil in a food processor until smooth.
- Season the shrimp with salt and pepper.
- Grill the shrimp over medium heat until pink and cooked through, about 2-3 minutes per side.
- Sauté the zucchini noodles in a pan with the remaining olive oil for 2-3 minutes.
- Toss the noodles with the pesto sauce.
- Top with grilled shrimp and serve immediately.

BREAKFAST :

DAY 3

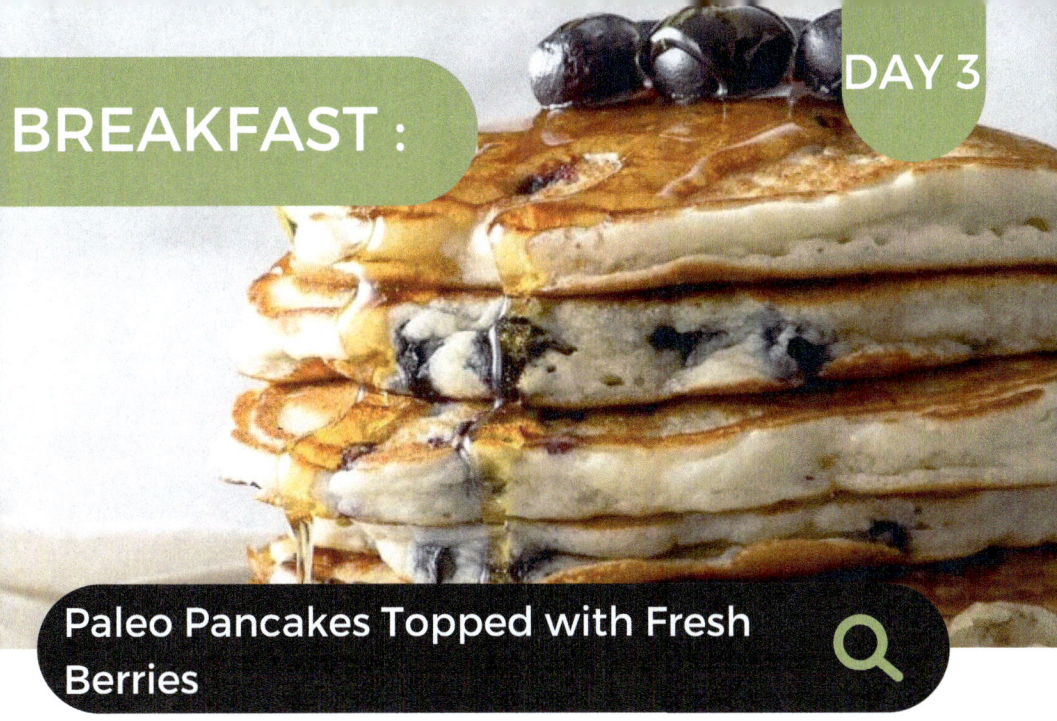

Paleo Pancakes Topped with Fresh Berries

INGREDIENTS

- 2 large eggs
- 1/2 banana, mashed
- 1/4 cup almond flour
- 1/4 teaspoon baking powder
- 1/4 teaspoon cinnamon
- 1/2 cup mixed berries (like strawberries, blueberries)
- Coconut oil for cooking
- small portion of Maple Syrup

PROCEDURE

- In a bowl, whisk together eggs, mashed banana, almond flour, baking powder, and cinnamon until smooth.
- Heat a non-stick skillet over medium heat and add a little coconut oil.
- Pour small amounts of the batter onto the skillet to form pancakes.
- Cook for 2-3 minutes on each side or until golden brown.
- Serve the pancakes topped with fresh berries.

LUNCH :

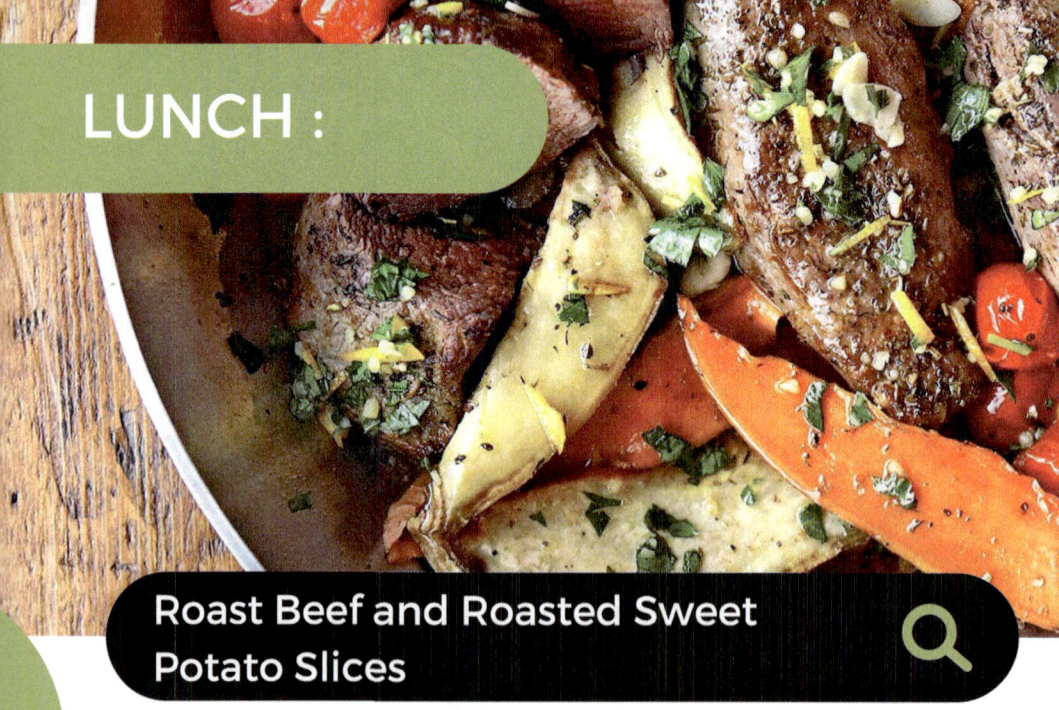

Roast Beef and Roasted Sweet Potato Slices

INGREDIENTS

- 1 small sweet potato, sliced into rounds
- 1/2 tablespoon olive oil
- Salt and pepper, to taste
- 4-5 slices of roast beef (ensure it's Paleo-friendly, without added sugars or preservatives)

PROCEDURE

- Preheat the oven to 400°F (200°C).
- Toss the sweet potato slices with olive oil, salt, and pepper.
- Spread the sweet potato slices in a single layer on a baking sheet.
- Roast in the oven for about 20-25 minutes, or until tender and slightly crisp.
- Serve the roasted sweet potato slices with the slices of roast beef.

PALEO DIET

DINNER :

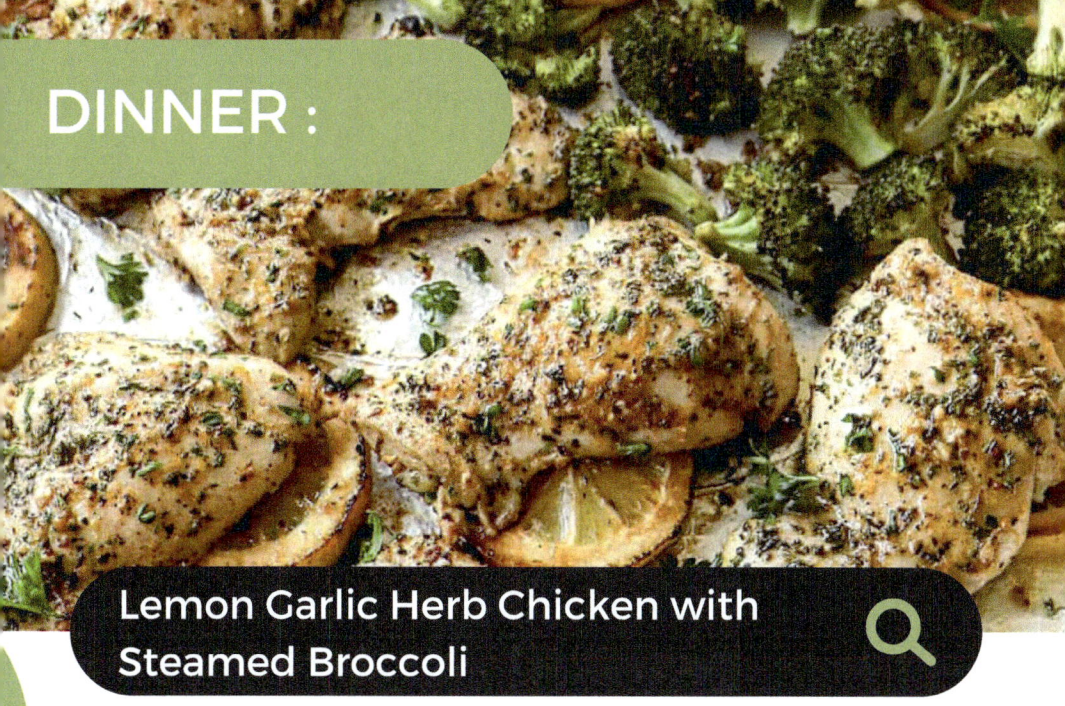

Lemon Garlic Herb Chicken with Steamed Broccoli

INGREDIENTS

- 1 chicken breast
- 1/2 lemon, juiced and zested
- 1 garlic clove, minced
- 1/2 tablespoon chopped fresh herbs (like parsley, rosemary)
- 1/2 tablespoon olive oil
- 1 cup broccoli florets
- Salt and pepper, to taste

PROCEDURE

- Marinate the chicken breast with lemon juice and zest, garlic, herbs, olive oil, salt, and pepper. Let it sit for at least 15 minutes.
- Preheat a grill or skillet over medium heat.
- Cook the chicken for about 6-7 minutes per side, or until fully cooked.
- While the chicken is cooking, steam the broccoli florets until tender, about 3-5 minutes.
- Serve the grilled chicken with the steamed broccoli.

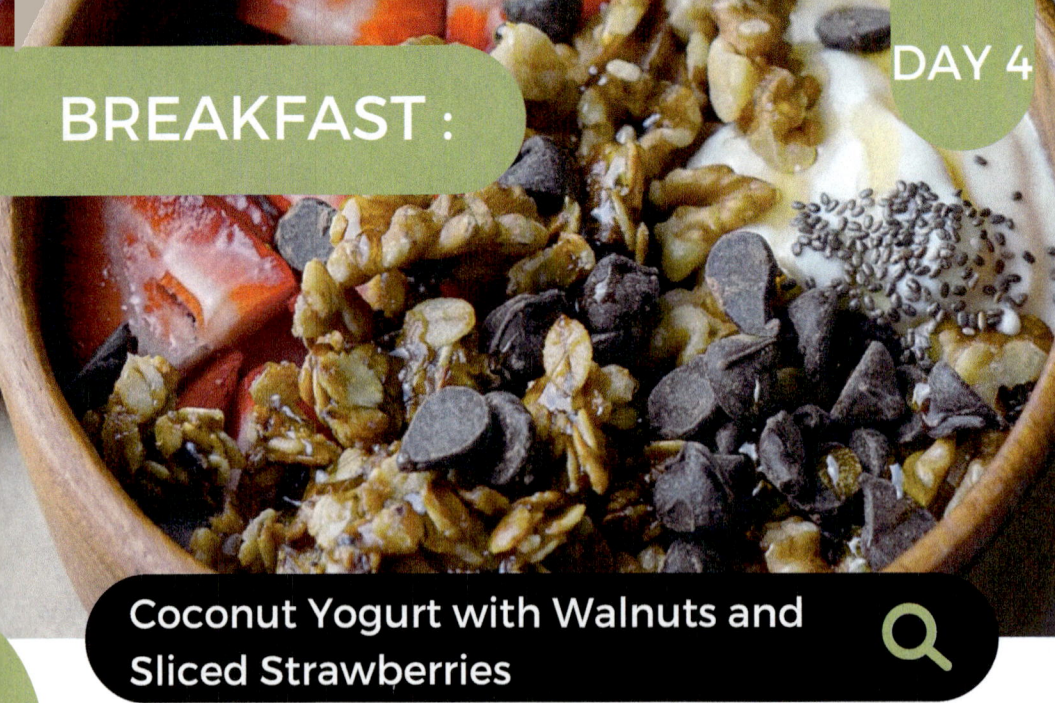

BREAKFAST :

DAY 4

Coconut Yogurt with Walnuts and Sliced Strawberries

INGREDIENTS

- 1 cup of coconut yogurt
- 1/2 cup sliced strawberries
- 1/4 cup chopped walnuts
- 1-2 tablespoons honey (optional)
- Fresh mint leaves (optional)

PROCEDURE

- Slice strawberries and chop walnuts.
- Layer coconut yogurt in a bowl or jar.
- Add sliced strawberries on top.
- Sprinkle chopped walnuts.
- Optionally, drizzle with honey.
- Garnish with fresh mint leaves if desired.
- Serve and enjoy!

PALEO DIET

LUNCH :

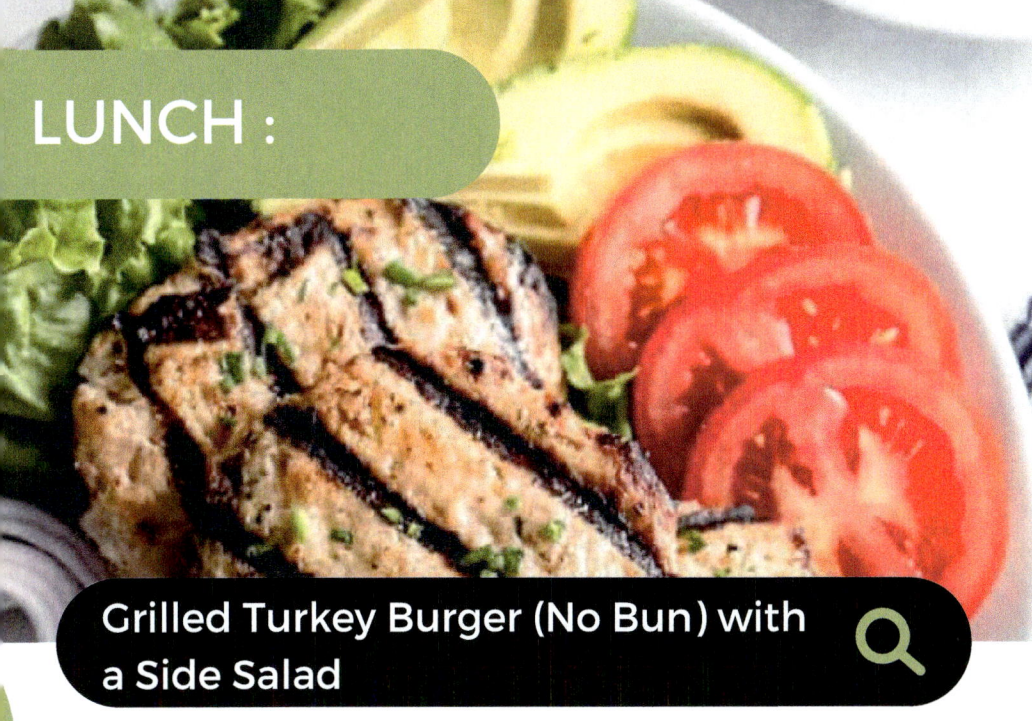

Grilled Turkey Burger (No Bun) with a Side Salad

INGREDIENTS

- 1 turkey burger patty (ensure it's Paleo-friendly, without added fillers)
- 2 cups mixed greens
- 1/4 cucumber, sliced
- 1/4 red bell pepper, sliced
- 1 tablespoon olive oil
- 1 teaspoon apple cider vinegar
- Salt and pepper, to taste

PROCEDURE

- Grill the turkey burger over medium heat until fully cooked, about 5-7 minutes per side.
- In a bowl, toss the mixed greens, cucumber, and bell pepper.
- In a small bowl, whisk together olive oil, apple cider vinegar, salt, and pepper to make a simple dressing.
- Dress the salad with the vinaigrette.
- Serve the grilled turkey burger alongside the fresh salad.

DINNER :

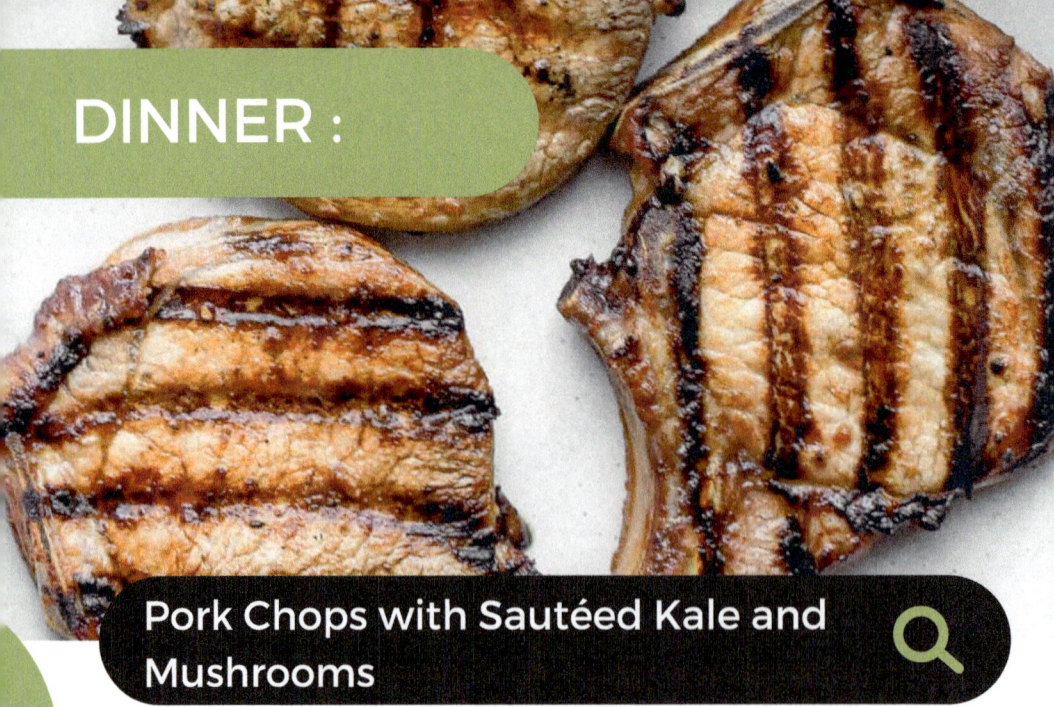

Pork Chops with Sautéed Kale and Mushrooms

INGREDIENTS

- 1 pork chop
- 1 cup kale, chopped
- 1/2 cup mushrooms, sliced
- 1 tablespoon olive oil
- 1 garlic clove, minced
- Salt and pepper, to taste

PROCEDURE

- Season the pork chop with salt and pepper.
- Heat a skillet over medium heat and add half of the olive oil.
- Cook the pork chop for about 5-7 minutes per side or until it reaches your desired doneness.
- In another skillet, heat the remaining olive oil. Add garlic, kale, and mushrooms, and sauté until the kale is wilted and mushrooms are browned, about 5-6 minutes.
- Season the vegetables with salt and pepper.
- Serve the pork chop with the sautéed kale and mushrooms.

PALEO DIET

BREAKFAST :

DAY 5

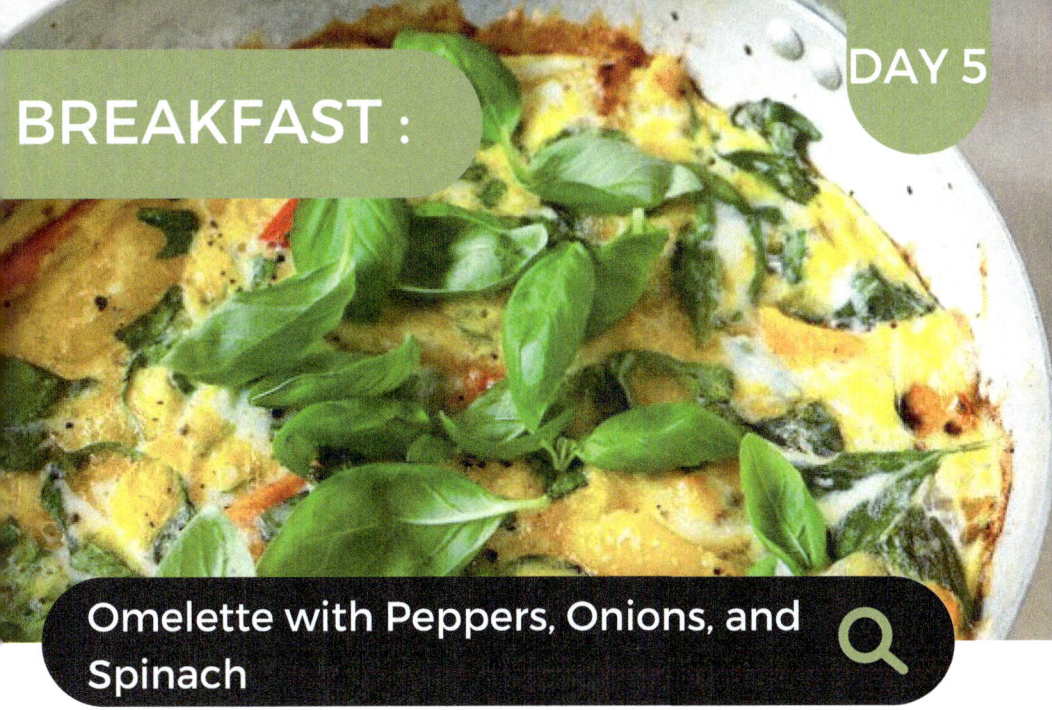

Omelette with Peppers, Onions, and Spinach

INGREDIENTS

- 2 large eggs
- 1/4 cup bell pepper, diced
- 1/4 cup onion, diced
- 1/2 cup fresh spinach, chopped
- 1 tablespoon olive oil
- Salt and pepper, to taste

PROCEDURE

- Beat the eggs in a bowl and season with salt and pepper.
- Heat the olive oil in a skillet over medium heat.
- Sauté the bell pepper and onion until they are soft, about 3-4 minutes.
- Add the spinach and cook until it wilts, about 1-2 minutes.
- Pour the beaten eggs over the vegetables.
- Cook without stirring for a few minutes until the bottom of the omelette sets.
- Carefully fold the omelette in half and cook for another minute.
- Serve the omelette hot.

PALEO DIET

LUNCH :

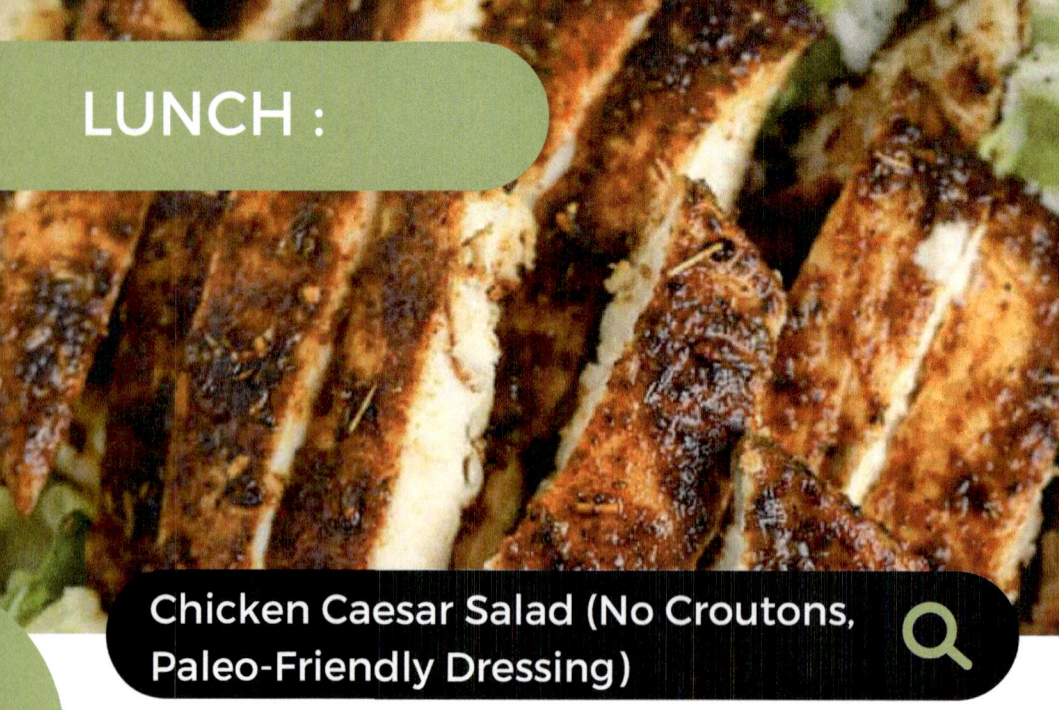

Chicken Caesar Salad (No Croutons, Paleo-Friendly Dressing)

INGREDIENTS

- 1 small chicken breast, grilled and sliced
- 2 cups Romaine lettuce, chopped
- 1/4 cup Paleo-friendly Caesar dressing (homemade or store-bought)
- 1 tablespoon grated Parmesan cheese (optional, omit for strict Paleo)

PROCEDURE

- In a large bowl, toss the chopped Romaine lettuce with the Caesar dressing.
- Top the salad with the sliced grilled chicken.
- If using, sprinkle with Parmesan cheese.
- Serve immediately for a fresh and satisfying meal.

PALEO DIET

DINNER:

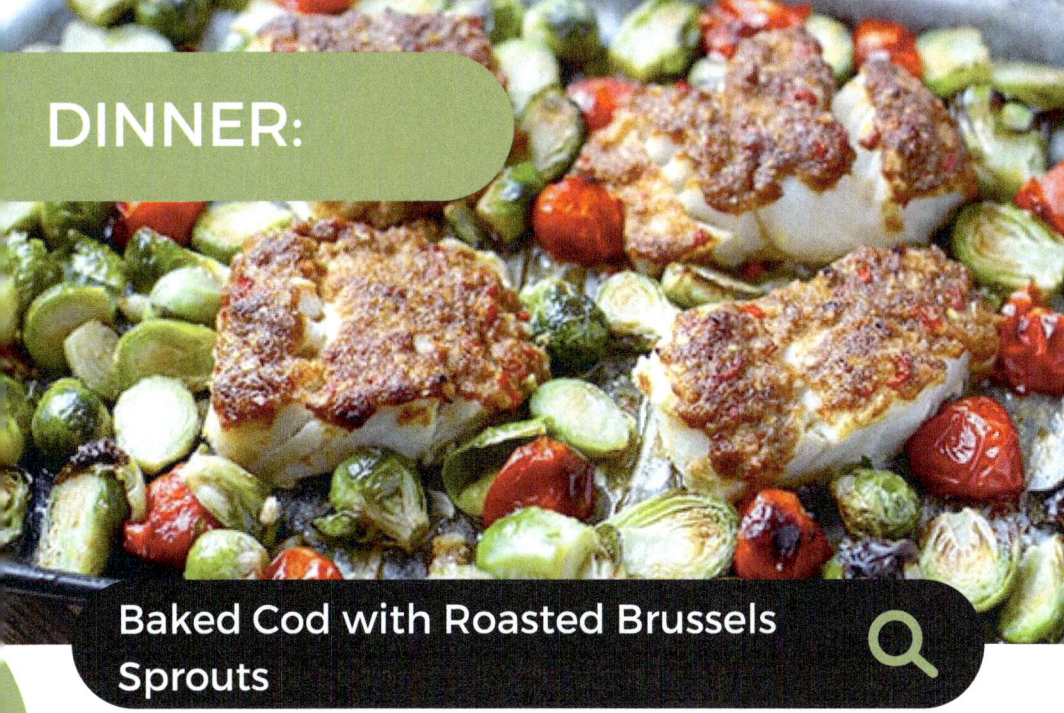

Baked Cod with Roasted Brussels Sprouts

INGREDIENTS

- 1 cod fillet (about 6 oz)
- 1 cup Brussels sprouts, halved
- 1 tablespoon olive oil
- 1/2 lemon, juiced
- Salt and pepper, to taste

PROCEDURE

- Preheat the oven to 400°F (200°C).
- Toss the Brussels sprouts with half of the olive oil, salt, and pepper, and spread them on a baking sheet.
- Bake for 15-20 minutes, or until tender and slightly browned.
- Meanwhile, season the cod with salt, pepper, and lemon juice.
- Heat the remaining olive oil in a skillet over medium heat and cook the cod for about 4-5 minutes per side, or until cooked through.
- Serve the baked cod alongside the roasted Brussels sprouts.

PALEO DIET

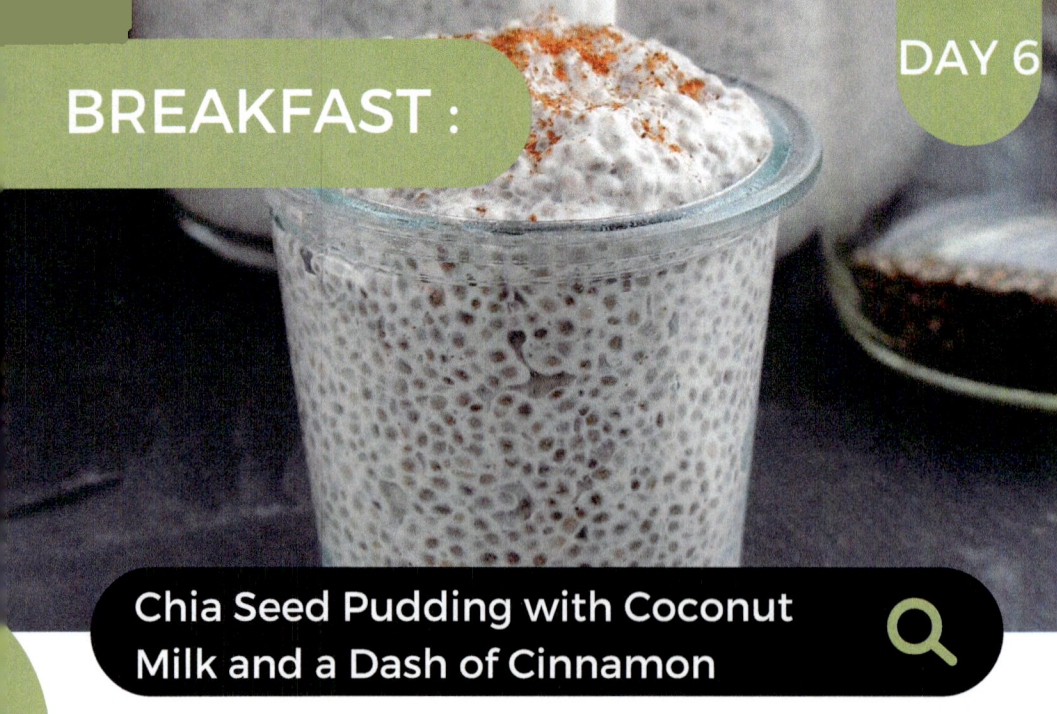

BREAKFAST :

DAY 6

Chia Seed Pudding with Coconut Milk and a Dash of Cinnamon

INGREDIENTS

- 3 tablespoons chia seeds
- 3/4 cup coconut milk (unsweetened)
- 1/2 teaspoon vanilla extract (optional)
- 1/4 teaspoon cinnamon
- 1 teaspoon honey or maple syrup (optional)

PROCEDURE

- In a bowl, mix the chia seeds with coconut milk, vanilla extract (if using), cinnamon, and honey or maple syrup (if using).
- Stir well to combine.
- Cover the bowl and refrigerate for at least 2 hours, preferably overnight, until the mixture achieves a pudding-like consistency.
- Stir again before serving. Add more coconut milk if it's too thick.

LUNCH :

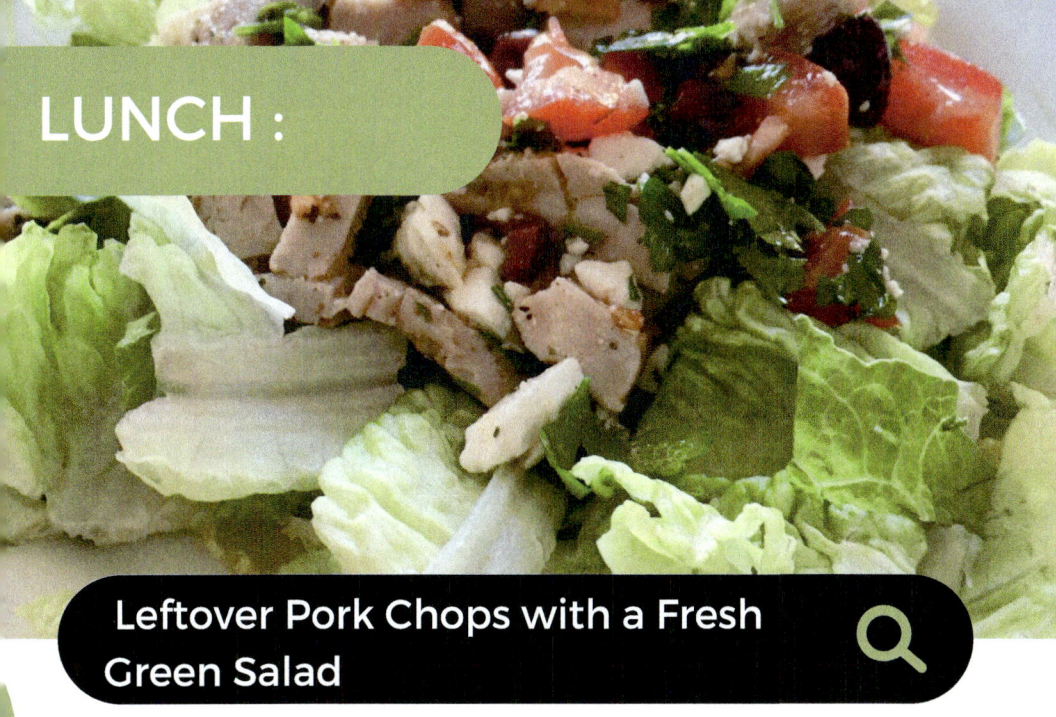

Leftover Pork Chops with a Fresh Green Salad

INGREDIENTS

- 1 leftover pork chop, reheated
- 2 cups mixed greens (like lettuce, arugula, spinach)
- 1/4 cucumber, sliced
- 1/4 carrot, shredded
- 2 tablespoons olive oil
- 1 tablespoon apple cider vinegar
- Salt and pepper, to taste

PROCEDURE

- In a large bowl, combine the mixed greens, cucumber, and carrot.
- In a small bowl, whisk together the olive oil, apple cider vinegar, salt, and pepper to create a simple dressing.
- Toss the salad with the dressing.
- Serve the salad with the reheated pork chop.

PALEO DIET

DINNER :

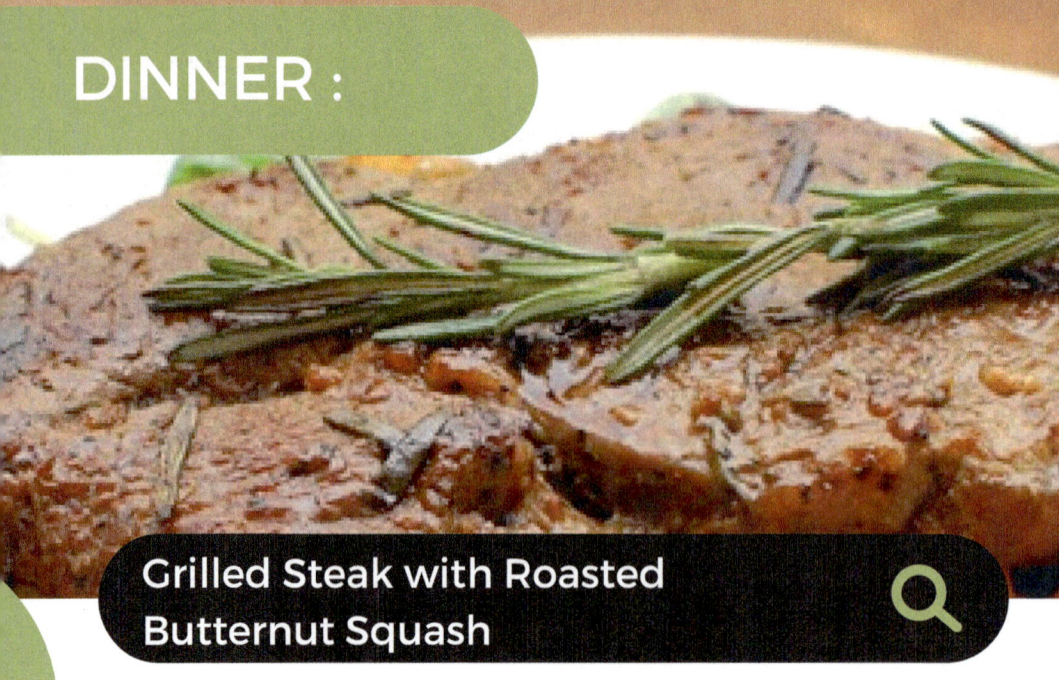

Grilled Steak with Roasted Butternut Squash

INGREDIENTS

- 1 steak cut of your choice (about 6 oz)
- 1 cup butternut squash, peeled and cubed
- 1 tablespoon olive oil
- Salt and pepper, to taste
- 1/2 teaspoon garlic powder (optional)

PROCEDURE

- Preheat the oven to 400°F (200°C).
- Toss the butternut squash cubes with half of the olive oil, salt, pepper, and garlic powder.
- Spread the squash on a baking sheet and roast for about 25-30 minutes, or until tender and slightly caramelized.
- Season the steak with salt and pepper.
- Grill the steak over medium-high heat to your preferred level of doneness, about 4-5 minutes per side for medium-rare.
- Let the steak rest for a few minutes before slicing.
- Serve the grilled steak alongside the roasted butternut squash.

PALEO DIET

BREAKFAST :

DAY 7

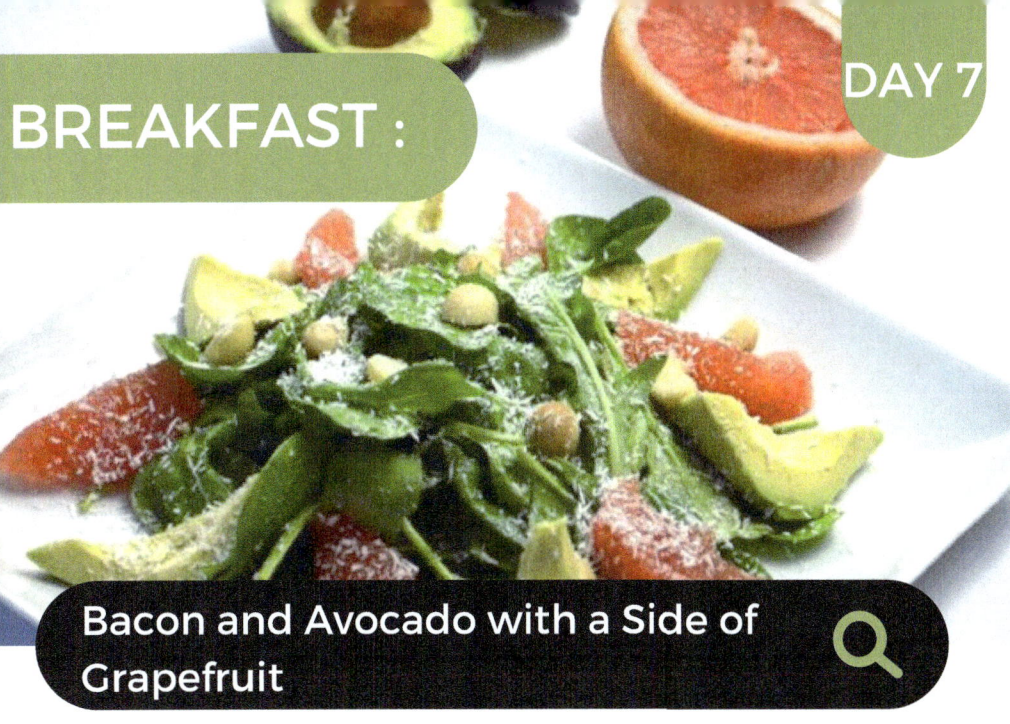

Bacon and Avocado with a Side of Grapefruit

INGREDIENTS

- 2 slices of bacon
- 1/2 ripe avocado
- 1/2 grapefruit

PROCEDURE

- Cook the bacon in a skillet over medium heat until crispy, about 4-5 minutes per side. Drain on a paper towel.
- Slice the avocado.
- Cut the grapefruit into segments.
- Serve the cooked bacon with avocado slices and grapefruit on the side.

PALEO DIET

LUNCH :

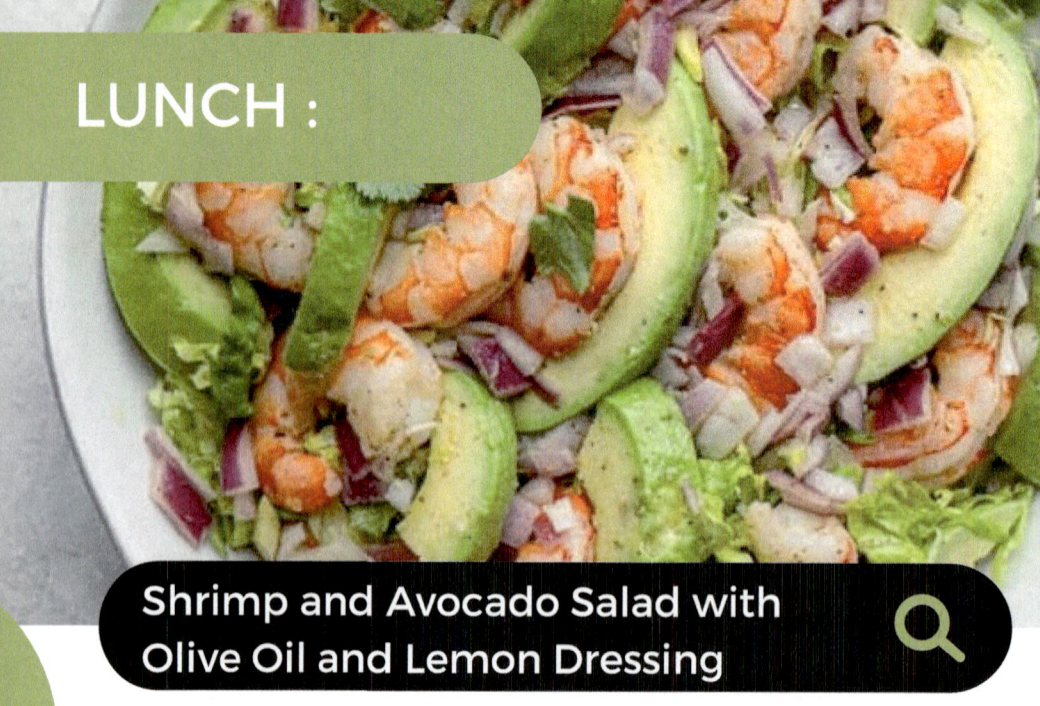

Shrimp and Avocado Salad with Olive Oil and Lemon Dressing

INGREDIENTS

- 5-6 large shrimp, peeled and deveined
- 1/2 ripe avocado, diced
- 2 cups mixed greens
- 1 tablespoon olive oil
- 1 tablespoon lemon juice
- Salt and pepper, to taste

PROCEDURE

- Season the shrimp with salt and pepper.
- Cook the shrimp in a skillet over medium heat until pink and opaque, about 2-3 minutes per side.
- In a bowl, combine the mixed greens and diced avocado.
- Whisk together olive oil and lemon juice for the dressing, and season with salt and pepper.
- Toss the salad with the dressing.
- Top the salad with the cooked shrimp.
- Serve immediately.

PALEO DIET

DINNER :

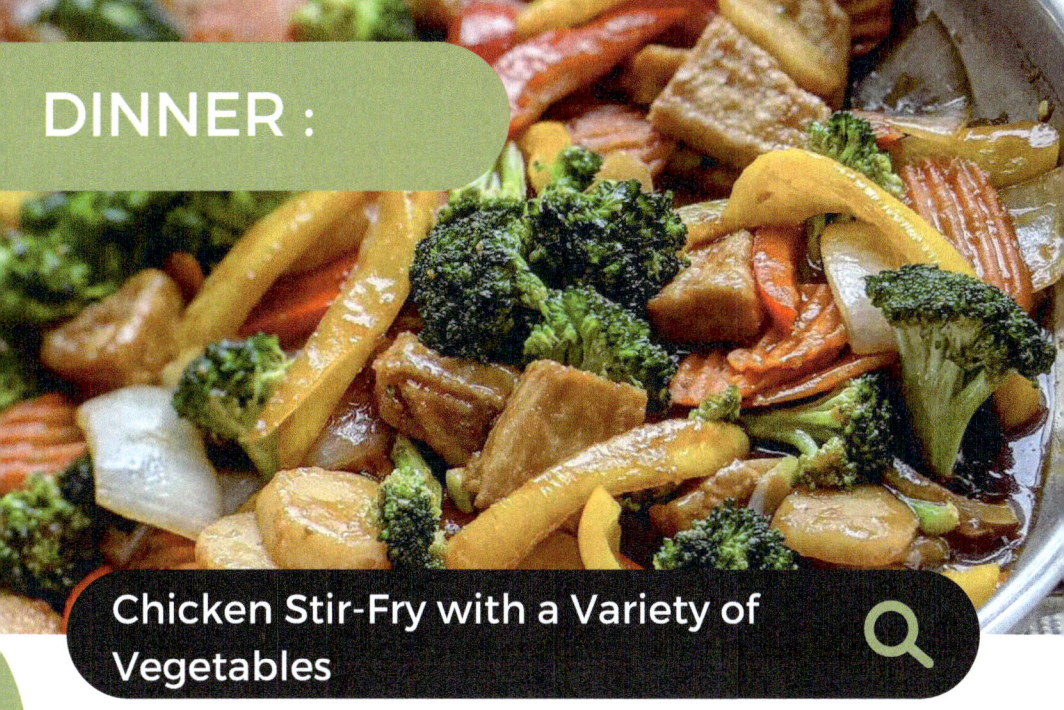

Chicken Stir-Fry with a Variety of Vegetables

INGREDIENTS

- 1 small chicken breast, thinly sliced
- 1/2 cup bell peppers, sliced
- 1/2 cup broccoli florets
- 1/4 cup onion, sliced
- 1 tablespoon coconut oil
- 1 garlic clove, minced
- 1 tablespoon soy sauce or coconut aminos
- Salt and pepper, to taste

PROCEDURE

- Heat the coconut oil in a wok or large skillet over medium-high heat.
- Add the garlic and onion, and sauté for a minute.
- Add the chicken slices and cook until no longer pink, about 3-4 minutes.
- Add the bell peppers and broccoli, and stir-fry for another 3-4 minutes until the vegetables are tender but still crisp.
- Add the soy sauce or coconut aminos, and season with salt and pepper.
- Stir everything well to combine.
- Serve the stir-fry hot.

PALEO DIET

After completing Week 1, it's important to reflect on how your body has responded to the dietary changes. Use the following scale to rate your experiences in various aspects of your health and well-being. Rate each category from 1 to 10 (where 1 is 'no improvement' and 10 is 'significant improvement').

1. Digestive Comfort
- Question: How would you rate the overall comfort of your digestive system this week?
- Rating (1-10): _____

2. Energy Levels
- Question: How do you feel about your energy levels after following the meal plan for a week?
- Rating (1-10): _____

3. Sleep Quality
- Question: Have you noticed any changes in the quality of your sleep?
- Rating (1-10): _____

4. Mood and Mental Clarity
- Question: How has your mood and mental clarity been affected by the dietary changes?
- Rating (1-10): _____

5. Physical Comfort and Pain Levels
- Question: If you previously experienced any physical discomfort or pain, have you noticed any changes in its intensity or frequency?
- Rating (1-10): _____

6. Skin Health
- Question: Have there been any noticeable changes in your skin health/appearance?
- Rating (1-10): _____

7. Cravings and Appetite Control
- Question: How would you rate your control over cravings and appetite this week?
- Rating (1-10): _____

8. Overall Well-being
- Question: Considering all factors, how would you rate your overall well-being after Week 1?
- Rating (1-10): _____

WEEK 1

DIGESTIVE COMFORT	1	2	3	4	5	6	7	8	9	10
ENERGY LEVELS	1	2	3	4	5	6	7	8	9	10
SLEEP QUALITY	1	2	3	4	5	6	7	8	9	10
MOOD & MENTAL CLARITY	1	2	3	4	5	6	7	8	9	10
PHYSICAL COMFORT	1	2	3	4	5	6	7	8	9	10
SKIN HEALTH	1	2	3	4	5	6	7	8	9	10
CRAVINGS CONTROL	1	2	3	4	5	6	7	8	9	10
OVERALL WELL-BEING	1	2	3	4	5	6	7	8	9	10

notes

....
....
....
....
....
....
....
....
....

PALEO DIET

FOR SPECIAL
notes

PALEO DIET

WEEK 2: EXPLORING DIVERSITY

As you step into Week 2, get ready to explore a diverse range of flavors and ingredients. This week is about broadening your Paleo palate and discovering the variety that this diet has to offer. Experiment with different recipes and find new favorites!

BREAKFAST :

DAY 8

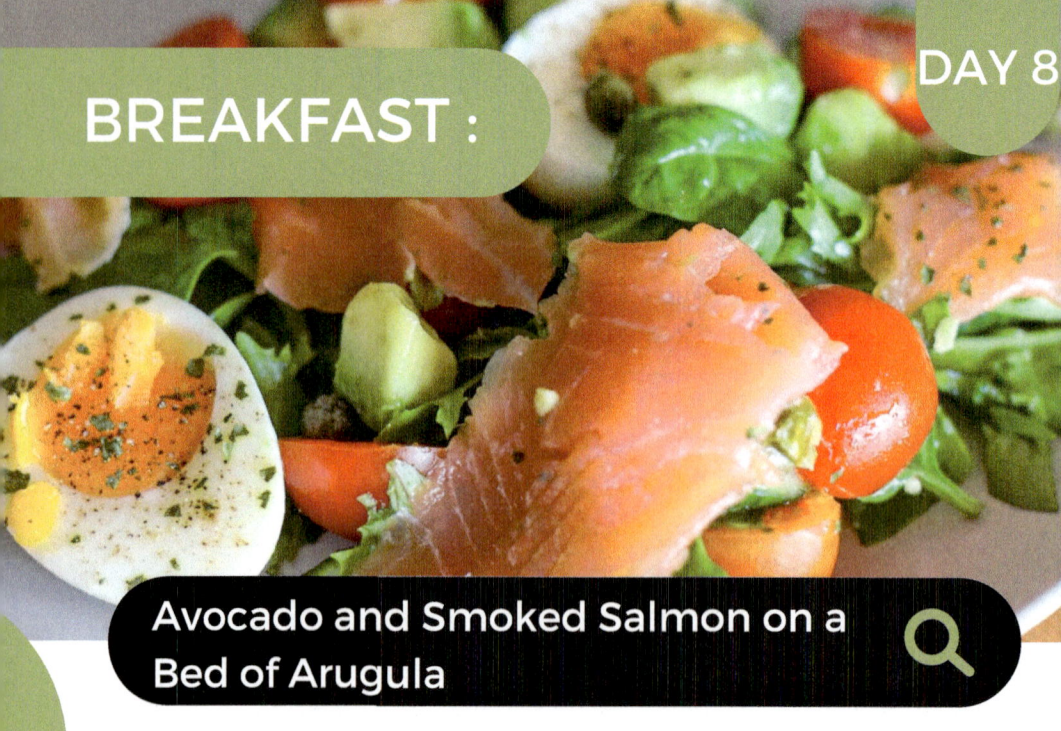

Avocado and Smoked Salmon on a Bed of Arugula

INGREDIENTS

- 1/2 ripe avocado, sliced
- 2-3 slices of smoked salmon
- 1 cup arugula
- 1 teaspoon olive oil
- 1 teaspoon lemon juice
- Salt and pepper, to taste

PROCEDURE

- Arrange the arugula on a plate.
- Drizzle the arugula with olive oil and lemon juice, then season lightly with salt and pepper.
- Lay the smoked salmon slices over the arugula.
- Add the sliced avocado on top.
- Serve immediately for a refreshing and nutritious breakfast.

LUNCH :

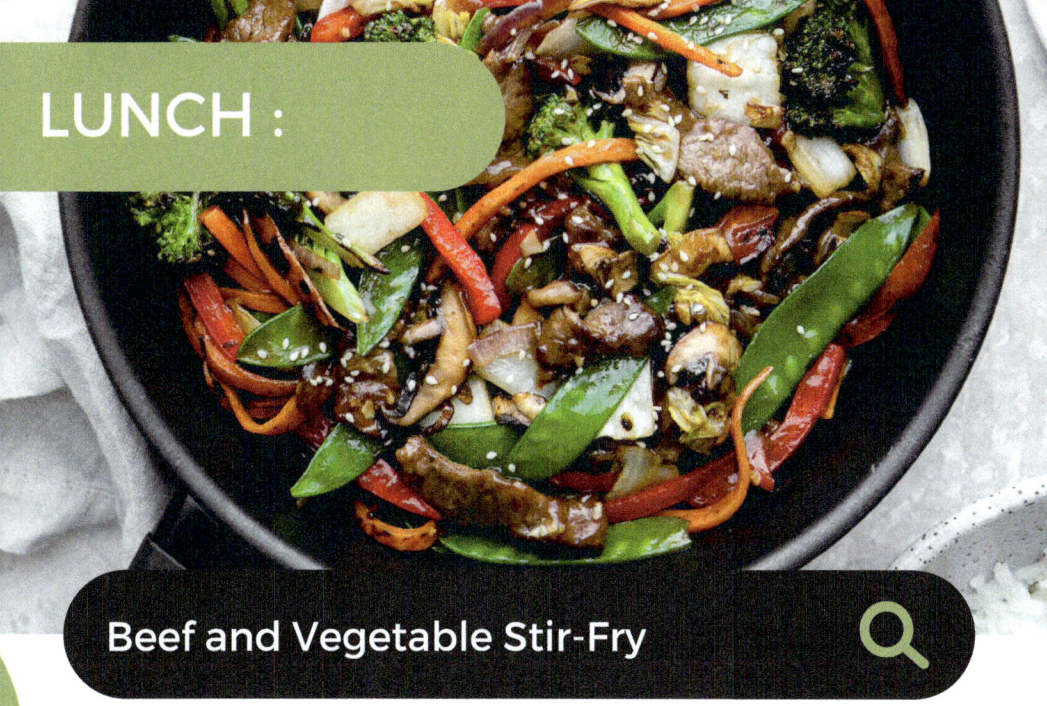

Beef and Vegetable Stir-Fry

INGREDIENTS

- 1 small beef steak (about 6 oz), thinly sliced
- 1/2 cup broccoli florets
- 1/2 bell pepper, sliced
- 1/4 onion, sliced
- 1 tablespoon coconut oil
- 1 garlic clove, minced
- 1 tablespoon soy sauce or coconut aminos
- Salt and pepper, to taste

PROCEDURE

- Heat the coconut oil in a wok or large skillet over medium-high heat.
- Add the garlic and onion, sautéing for a minute.
- Add the beef slices, cooking until they start to brown, about 3-4 minutes.
- Add the broccoli and bell pepper, continuing to stir-fry for another 3-4 minutes until the vegetables are tender but still crisp.
- Add soy sauce or coconut aminos, seasoning with salt and pepper.
- Stir everything together to combine.
- Serve the stir-fry hot.

PALEO DIET

DINNER :

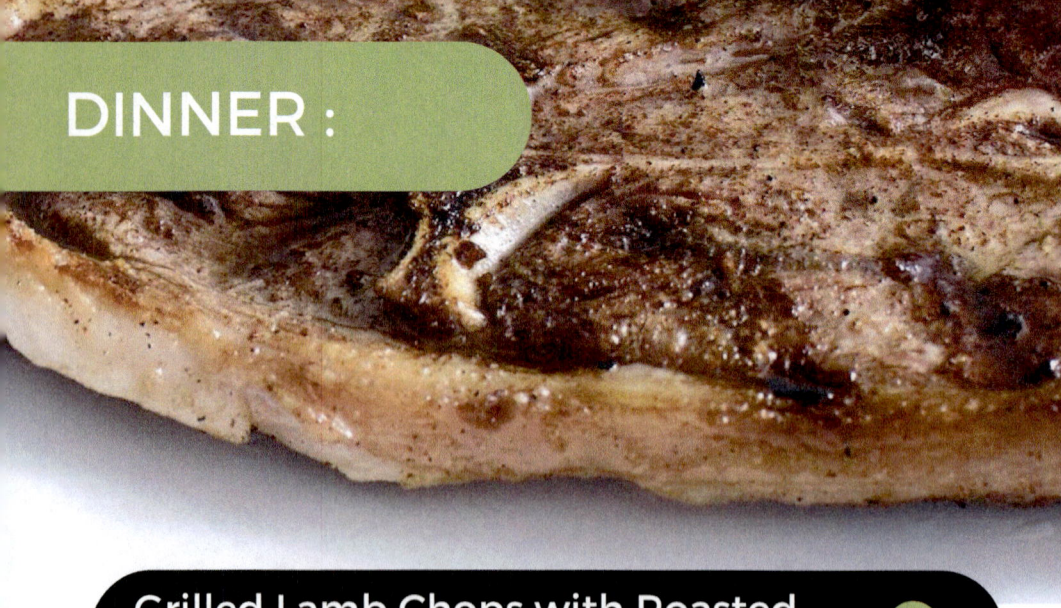

Grilled Lamb Chops with Roasted Cauliflower

INGREDIENTS

- 2 lamb chops
- 1 cup cauliflower florets
- 1 tablespoon olive oil
- 1/2 teaspoon garlic powder
- Salt and pepper, to taste

PROCEDURE

- Preheat the oven to 400°F (200°C).
- Toss the cauliflower florets with olive oil, garlic powder, salt, and pepper.
- Spread the cauliflower on a baking sheet and roast for about 20-25 minutes, until tender and golden.
- Season the lamb chops with salt and pepper.
- Grill the lamb chops over medium-high heat to your preferred level of doneness, about 3-4 minutes per side for medium-rare.
- Let the lamb chops rest for a few minutes before serving.
- Serve the grilled lamb chops alongside the roasted cauliflower.

PALEO DIET

BREAKFAST :

DAY 9

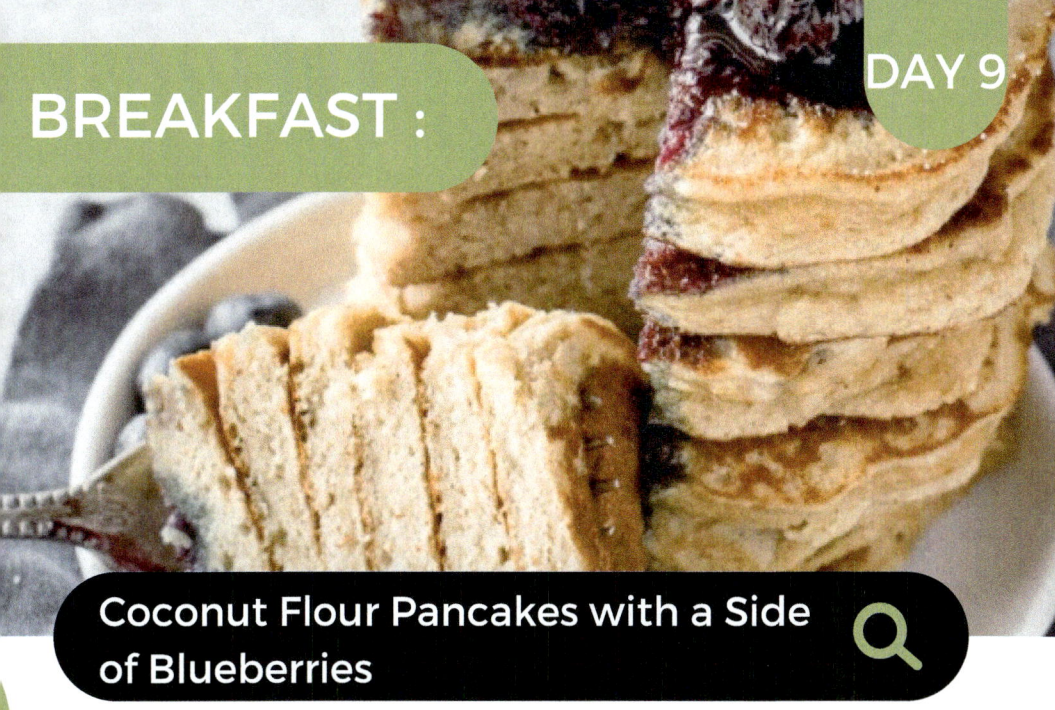

Coconut Flour Pancakes with a Side of Blueberries

INGREDIENTS

- 2 large eggs
- 1/4 cup coconut flour
- 1/4 cup almond milk (unsweetened)
- 1 tablespoon honey or maple syrup (optional)
- 1/2 teaspoon baking powder
- 1/4 teaspoon vanilla extract (optional)
- Coconut oil for cooking
- 1/2 cup blueberries

PROCEDURE

- In a bowl, whisk together eggs, almond milk, honey or maple syrup (if using), and vanilla extract.
- Add coconut flour and baking powder, mixing until smooth.
- Heat a skillet over medium heat and add a little coconut oil.
- Pour small amounts of the batter onto the skillet to form pancakes.
- Cook for 2-3 minutes on each side or until golden brown.
- Serve the pancakes with a side of blueberries.

PALEO DIET

LUNCH :

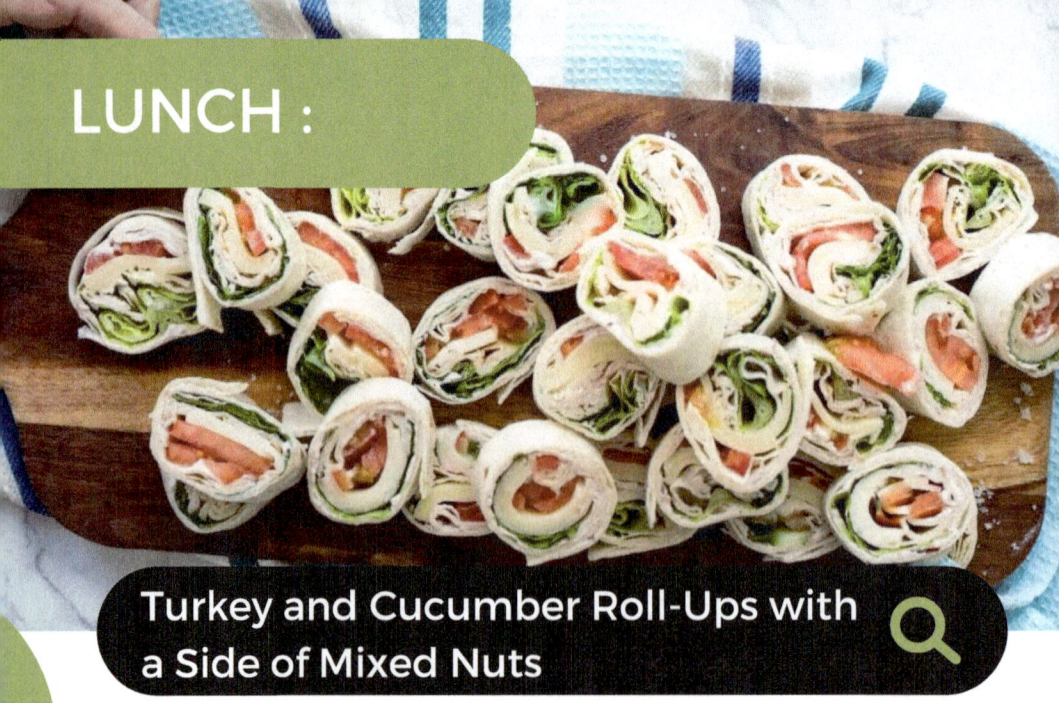

Turkey and Cucumber Roll-Ups with a Side of Mixed Nuts

INGREDIENTS

- 4-5 slices of turkey breast (ensure it's Paleo-friendly)
- 1/2 cucumber, thinly sliced lengthwise
- Mixed nuts (almonds, walnuts, cashews) - a small handful

PROCEDURE

- Lay out the turkey slices.
- Place a few cucumber slices on each turkey slice.
- Roll the turkey slices tightly around the cucumber.
- Serve with a side of mixed nuts.

PALEO DIET

DINNER :

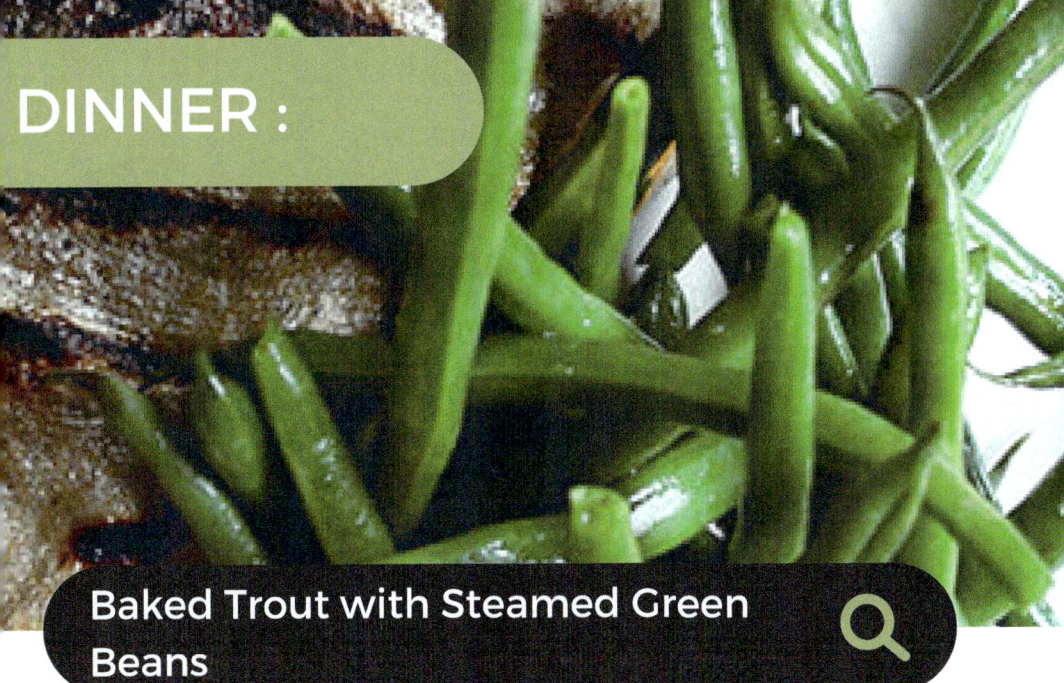

Baked Trout with Steamed Green Beans

INGREDIENTS

- 1 trout fillet (about 6 oz)
- 1 cup green beans, ends trimmed
- 1 tablespoon olive oil
- 1/2 lemon, juiced
- Salt and pepper, to taste

PROCEDURE

- Preheat the oven to 400°F (200°C).
- Place the trout fillet on a baking sheet.
- Drizzle with olive oil and lemon juice, and season with salt and pepper.
- Bake for 12-15 minutes, or until the trout is cooked through and flakes easily with a fork.
- Meanwhile, steam the green beans until tender, about 3-5 minutes.
- Serve the baked trout with the steamed green beans on the side.

PALEO DIET

BREAKFAST :

DAY10

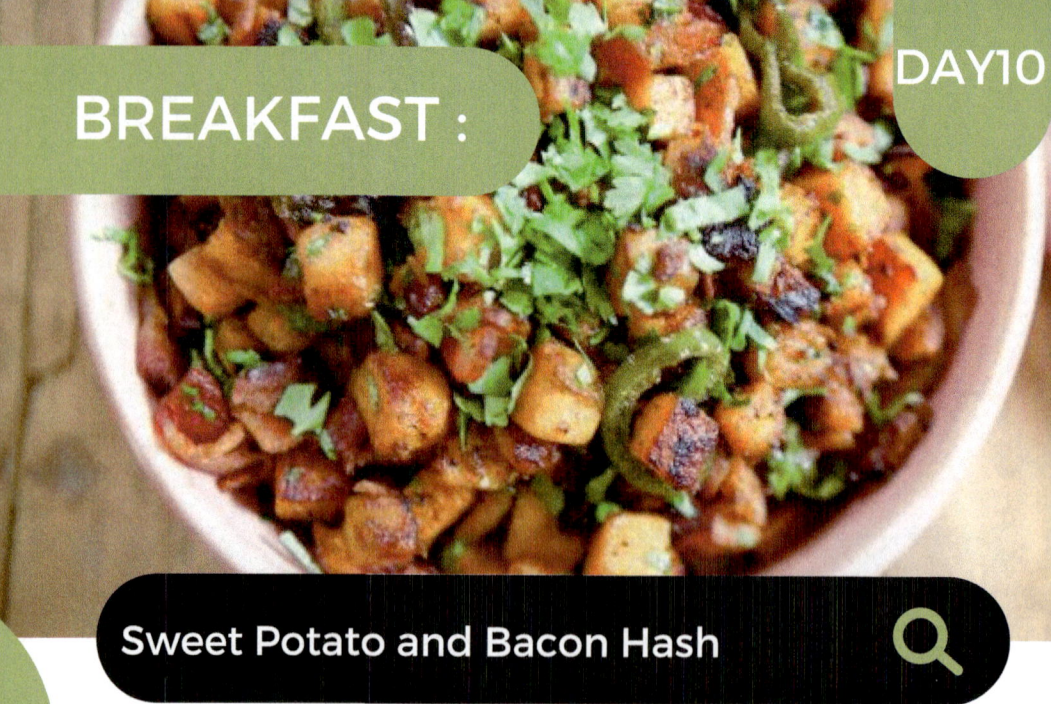

Sweet Potato and Bacon Hash

INGREDIENTS

- 1 medium sweet potato, peeled and diced
- 2 slices of bacon, chopped
- 1/4 onion, diced
- Salt and pepper, to taste
- 1 tablespoon olive oil (if needed)

PROCEDURE

- In a skillet, cook the bacon over medium heat until crispy. Remove and set aside, leaving the bacon fat in the skillet.
- Add the diced sweet potato to the skillet. If the bacon didn't render enough fat, add a tablespoon of olive oil.
- Cook the sweet potato for about 10 minutes, until tender and starting to brown.
- Add the diced onion to the skillet, and cook for another 5 minutes until the onion is soft and translucent.
- Return the cooked bacon to the skillet, mix with the sweet potato and onion, and season with salt and pepper.
- Serve hot as a hearty and flavorful breakfast.

PALEO DIET

LUNCH :

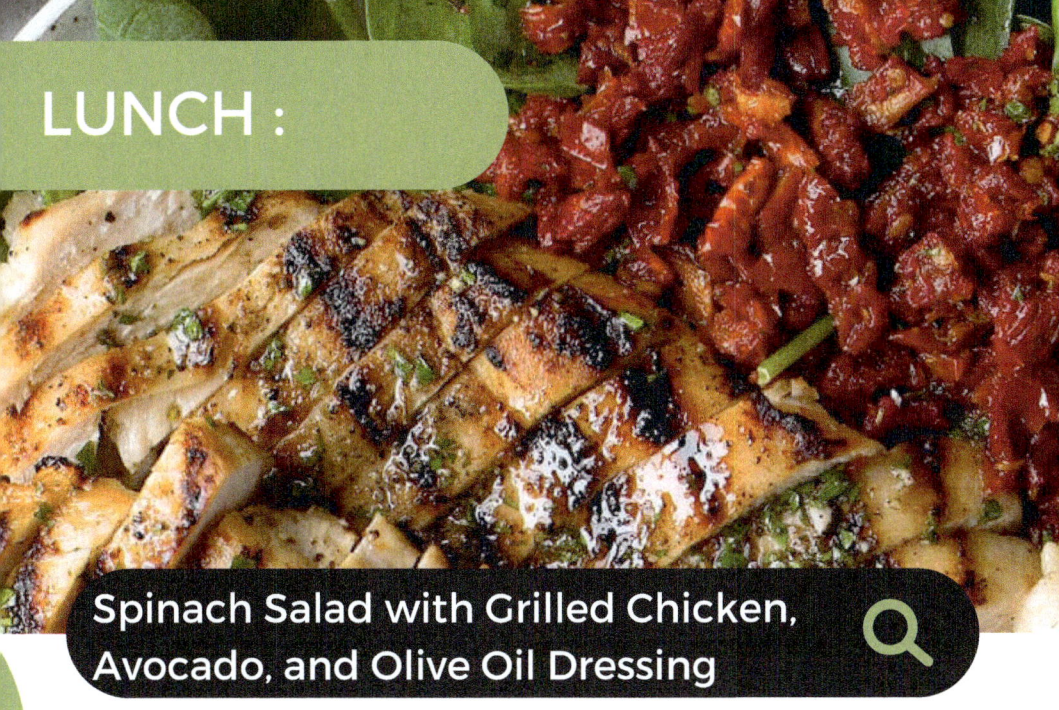

Spinach Salad with Grilled Chicken, Avocado, and Olive Oil Dressing

INGREDIENTS

- 1 small chicken breast, grilled and sliced
- 2 cups fresh spinach
- 1/2 avocado, sliced
- 2 tablespoons olive oil
- 1 tablespoon lemon juice
- Salt and pepper, to taste

PROCEDURE

- In a large bowl, place the fresh spinach and top with sliced avocado and grilled chicken.
- In a small bowl, whisk together olive oil, lemon juice, salt, and pepper to make a dressing.
- Drizzle the dressing over the salad.
- Toss gently to combine.
- Serve immediately for a fresh and nutritious lunch.

PALEO DIET

DINNER :

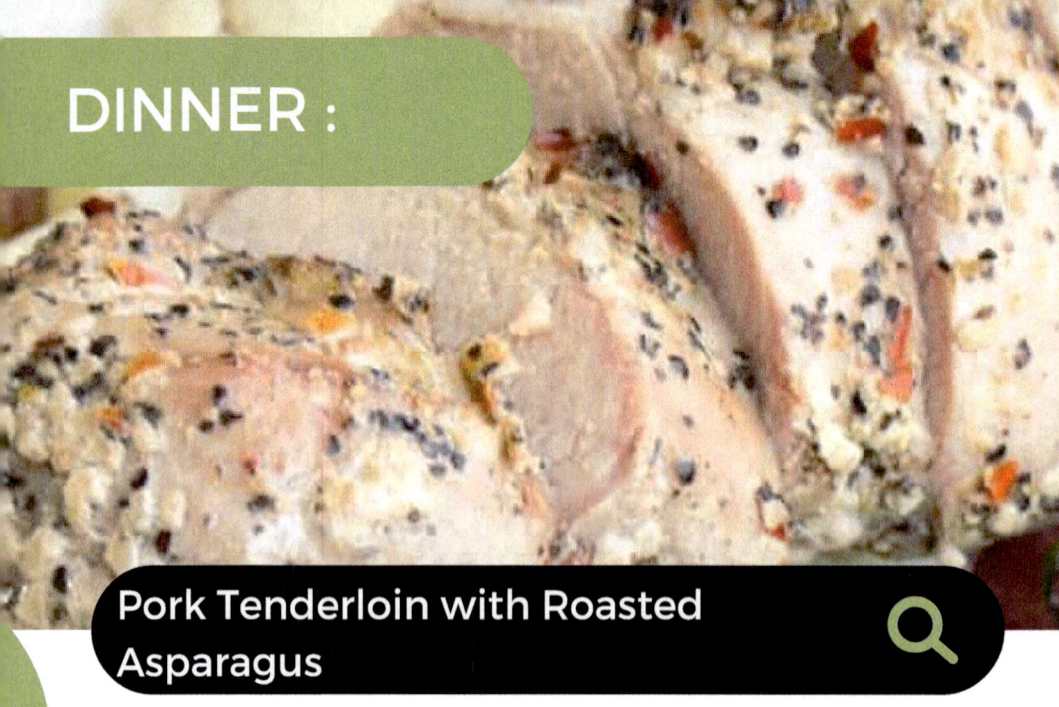

Pork Tenderloin with Roasted Asparagus

INGREDIENTS

- 1 pork tenderloin (about 6 oz)
- 1 cup asparagus spears, ends trimmed
- 1 tablespoon olive oil
- 1/2 teaspoon garlic powder
- Salt and pepper, to taste

PROCEDURE

- Preheat the oven to 375°F (190°C).
- Season the pork tenderloin with salt, pepper, and garlic powder.
- Place the pork in a baking dish.
- Toss the asparagus spears with olive oil, salt, and pepper, and arrange them around the pork in the dish.
- Roast in the preheated oven for about 20-25 minutes, or until the pork reaches an internal temperature of 145°F (63°C).
- Let the pork rest for a few minutes before slicing.
- Serve the pork tenderloin with the roasted asparagus.

BREAKFAST :

DAY 11

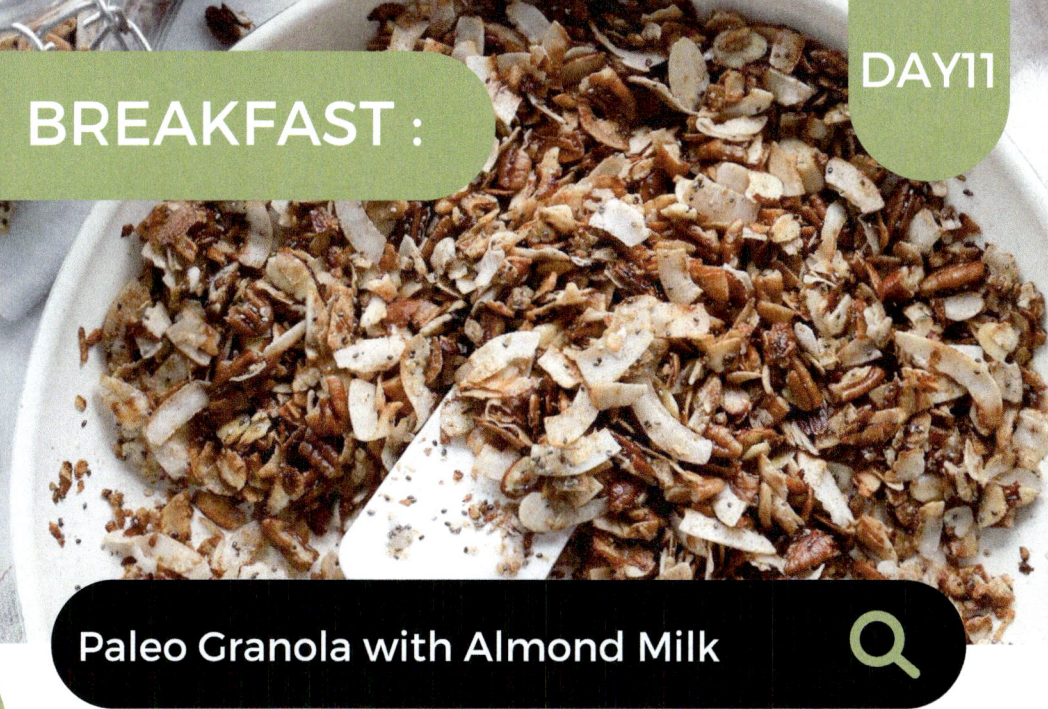

Paleo Granola with Almond Milk

INGREDIENTS

- 1/2 cup mixed nuts (almonds, walnuts, pecans), roughly chopped
- 1/4 cup pumpkin seeds
- 1/4 cup shredded coconut (unsweetened)
- 1 tablespoon honey or maple syrup
- 1/2 teaspoon cinnamon
- 1 tablespoon coconut oil, melted
- 3/4 cup almond milk (unsweetened)

PROCEDURE

- Preheat the oven to 300°F (150°C).
- In a bowl, mix together the nuts, pumpkin seeds, shredded coconut, honey or maple syrup, cinnamon, and melted coconut oil.
- Spread the mixture evenly on a baking sheet lined with parchment paper.
- Bake for about 15-20 minutes, stirring occasionally, until golden brown.
- Let the granola cool and become crisp.
- Serve with almond milk.

PALEO DIET

LUNCH :

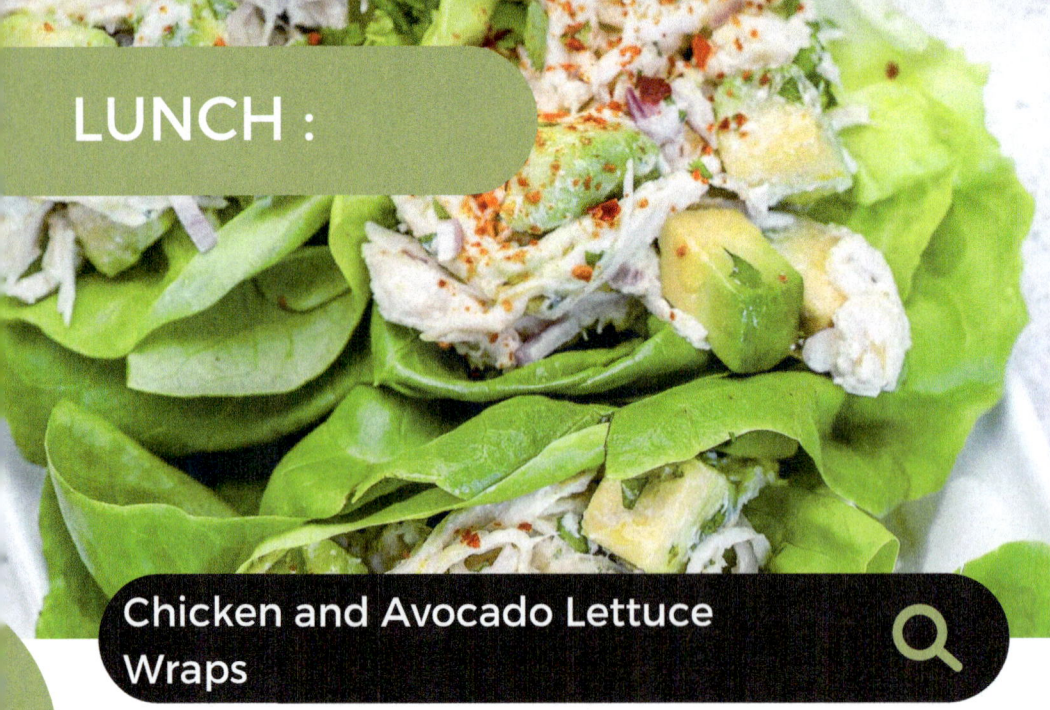

Chicken and Avocado Lettuce Wraps

INGREDIENTS

- 1 small chicken breast, cooked and shredded
- 1/2 ripe avocado, diced
- 2 large lettuce leaves (Romaine or Iceberg)
- Salt and pepper, to taste
- A squeeze of lemon juice (optional)

PROCEDURE

- In a bowl, mix the shredded chicken, diced avocado, salt, pepper, and lemon juice.
- Spoon the mixture onto the lettuce leaves.
- Roll up the lettuce leaves to form wraps.
- Serve immediately for a fresh and satisfying lunch.

PALEO DIET

DINNER:

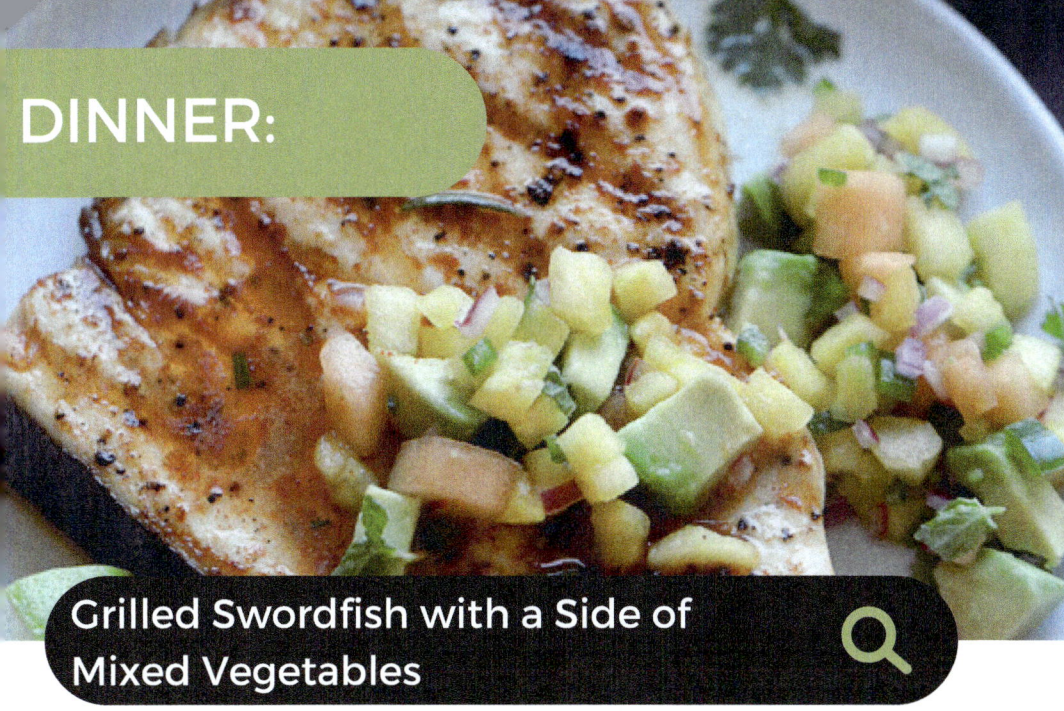

Grilled Swordfish with a Side of Mixed Vegetables

INGREDIENTS

- 1 swordfish steak (about 6 oz)
- 1 cup mixed vegetables (broccoli, carrots, bell peppers)
- 1 tablespoon olive oil
- Salt and pepper, to taste
- Lemon wedges, for serving

PROCEDURE

- Season the swordfish steak with salt and pepper.
- Grill the swordfish over medium heat until it's cooked through, about 3-4 minutes per side.
- Toss the mixed vegetables with olive oil, salt, and pepper.
- Grill or sauté the vegetables until tender-crisp, about 5-6 minutes.
- Serve the grilled swordfish with the mixed vegetables and a lemon wedge.

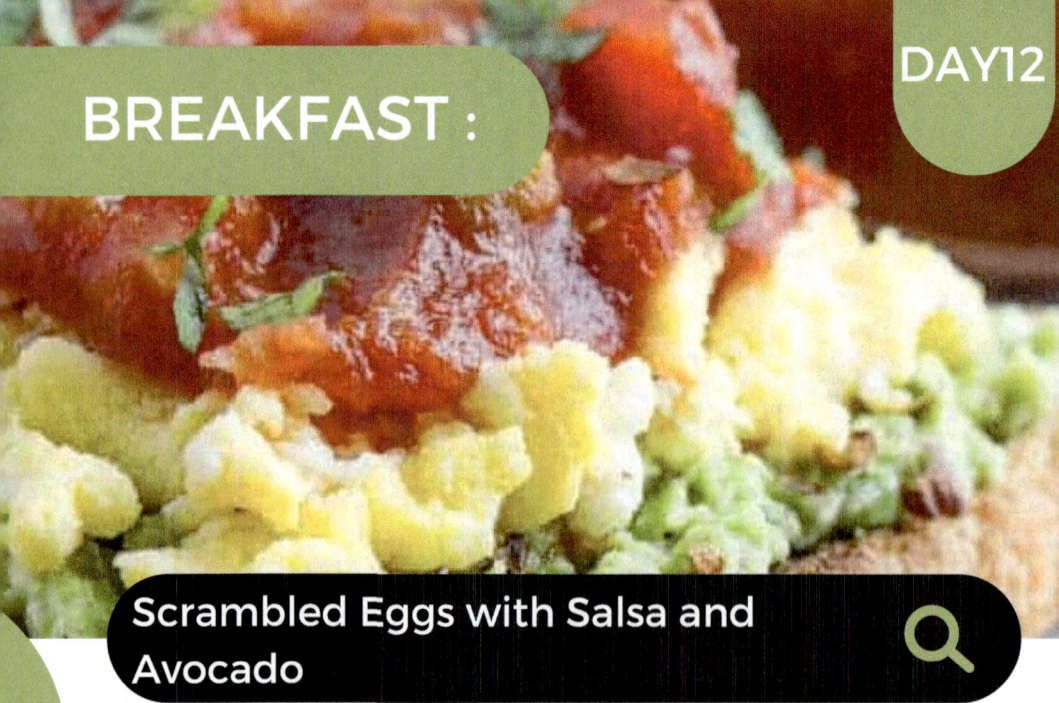

BREAKFAST :

DAY 12

Scrambled Eggs with Salsa and Avocado

INGREDIENTS

- 2 large eggs
- 1/2 ripe avocado, diced
- 2 tablespoons salsa (ensure it's Paleo-friendly)
- 1 tablespoon olive oil
- Salt and pepper, to taste

PROCEDURE

- Beat the eggs in a bowl and season with salt and pepper.
- Heat the olive oil in a skillet over medium heat.
- Pour the eggs into the skillet and scramble them until they are just set.
- Remove from heat and gently mix in the salsa.
- Serve the scrambled eggs with diced avocado on top.

LUNCH :

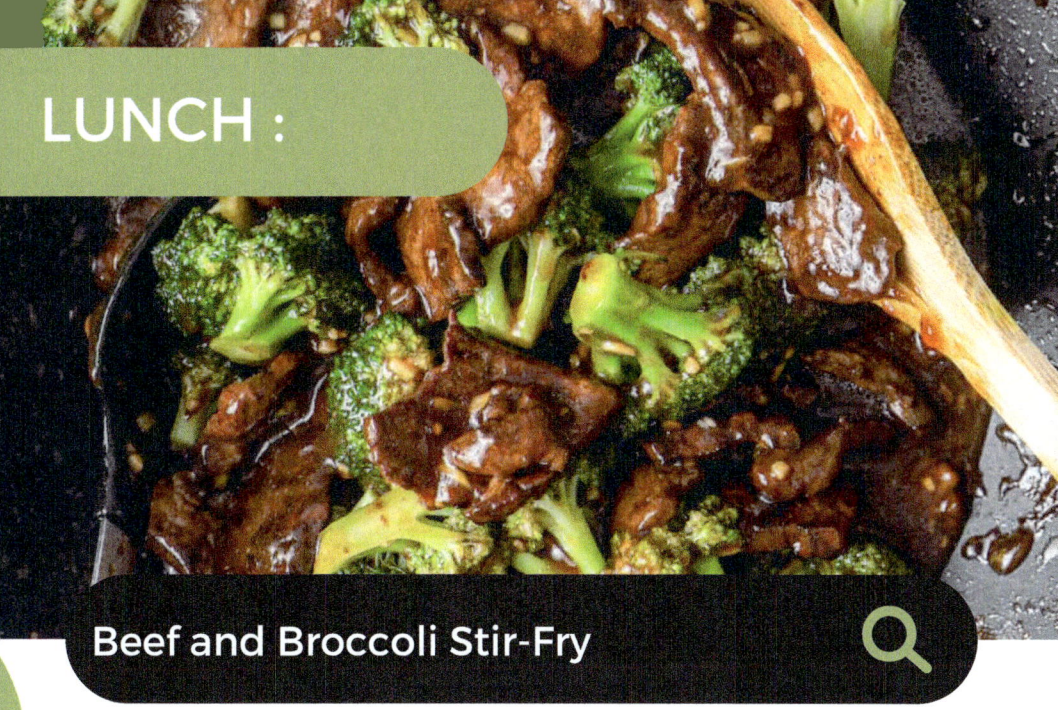

Beef and Broccoli Stir-Fry

INGREDIENTS

- 1 small beef steak (about 6 oz), thinly sliced
- 1 cup broccoli florets
- 1 tablespoon coconut oil
- 1 garlic clove, minced
- 1 tablespoon soy sauce or coconut aminos
- Salt and pepper, to taste

PROCEDURE

- Heat the coconut oil in a wok or large skillet over medium-high heat.
- Add the garlic and cook for about 30 seconds.
- Add the beef slices, cooking until they start to brown, about 3-4 minutes.
- Add the broccoli and continue to stir-fry until the broccoli is tender but still crisp, about 3-4 minutes.
- Add soy sauce or coconut aminos, seasoning with salt and pepper.
- Stir everything together to combine.
- Serve the stir-fry hot.

PALEO DIET

DINNER :

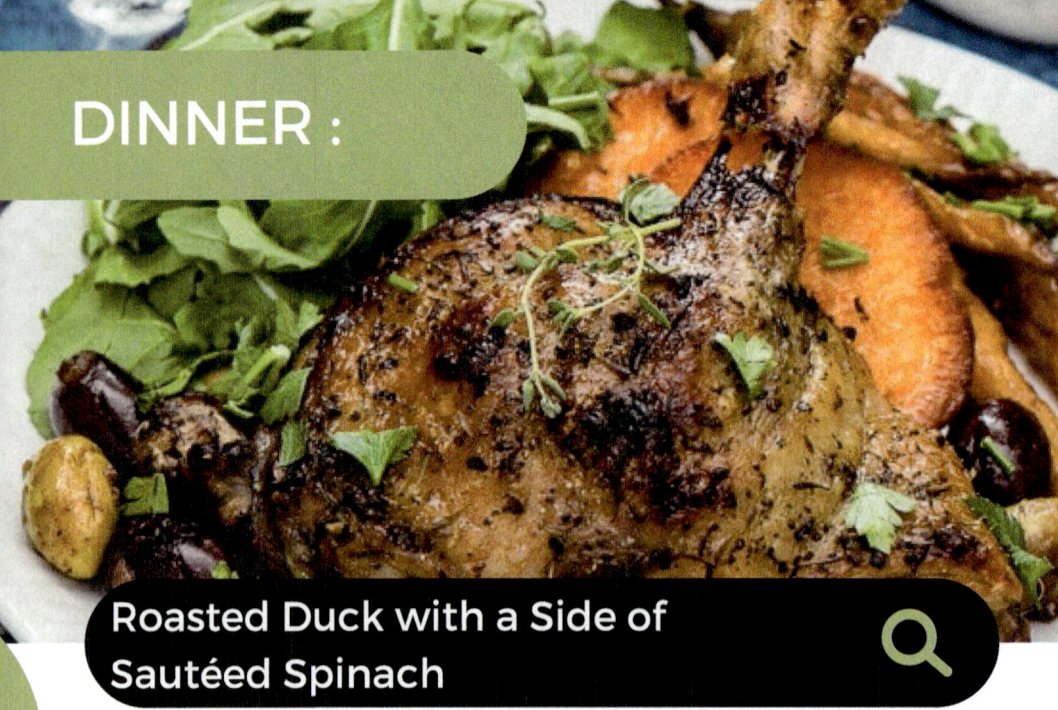

Roasted Duck with a Side of Sautéed Spinach

INGREDIENTS

- 1 duck breast
- Salt and pepper, to taste
- 1 cup spinach
- 1 tablespoon olive oil
- 1 garlic clove, minced

PROCEDURE

- Preheat the oven to 400°F (200°C).
- Score the skin of the duck breast and season both sides with salt and pepper.
- Place the duck breast skin-side down in a cold skillet. Turn the heat to medium and cook until the skin is crispy, about 6-8 minutes.
- Transfer the duck, skin-side up, to a baking dish and roast in the oven for about 6-10 minutes (depending on desired doneness).
- While the duck is roasting, heat olive oil in a skillet over medium heat.
- Add minced garlic and sauté for 30 seconds.
- Add the spinach and sauté until wilted, about 2-3 minutes.
- Season the spinach with salt and pepper.
- Slice the duck and serve with the sautéed spinach.

PALEO DIET

BREAKFAST :

DAY13

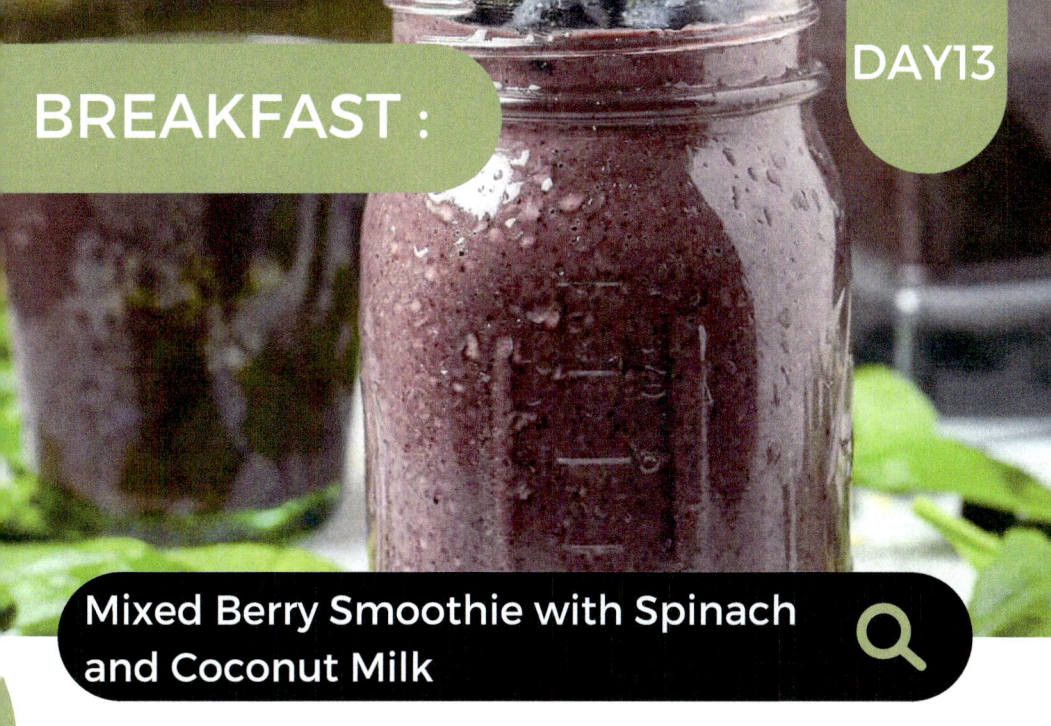

Mixed Berry Smoothie with Spinach and Coconut Milk

INGREDIENTS

- 1/2 cup mixed berries (like strawberries, blueberries, raspberries)
- 1 cup spinach
- 3/4 cup coconut milk (unsweetened)
- 1 tablespoon chia seeds (optional)
- Ice cubes (optional)

PROCEDURE

- Combine the mixed berries, spinach, coconut milk, and chia seeds (if using) in a blender.
- Add ice cubes if you prefer a colder smoothie.
- Blend until smooth and creamy.
- Serve immediately in a tall glass.

LUNCH :

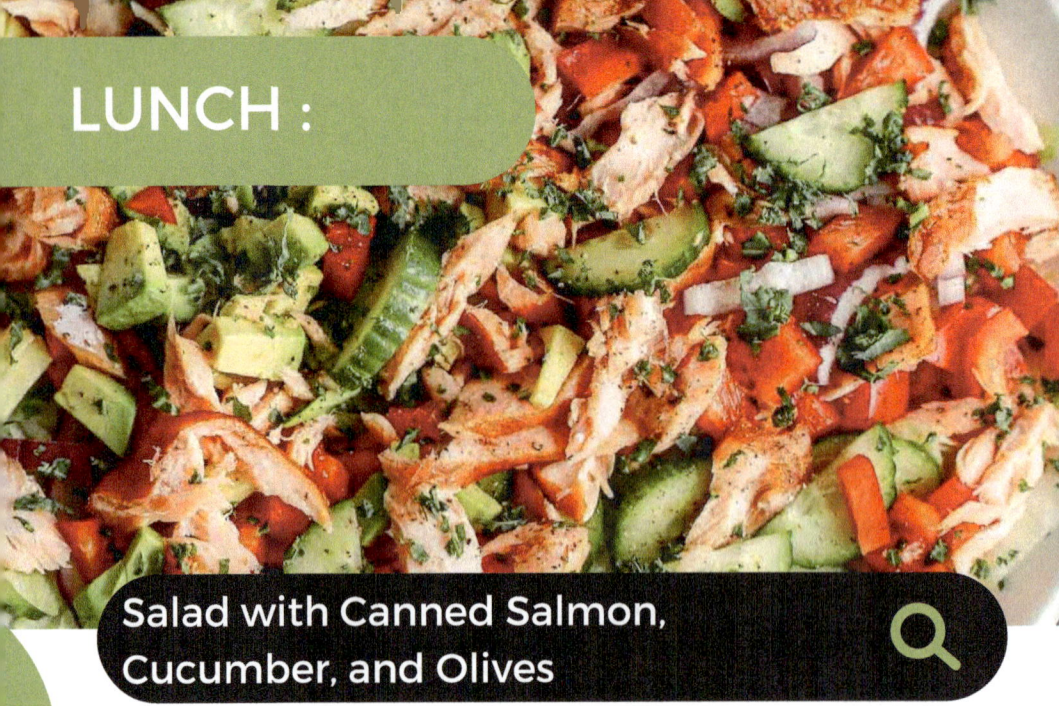

Salad with Canned Salmon, Cucumber, and Olives

INGREDIENTS

- 1 can of salmon (about 4 oz), drained
- 2 cups mixed greens
- 1/2 cucumber, sliced
- 1/4 cup olives, pitted
- 2 tablespoons olive oil
- 1 tablespoon lemon juice
- Salt and pepper, to taste

PROCEDURE

- In a large bowl, place the mixed greens.
- Top the greens with the canned salmon, cucumber slices, and olives.
- In a small bowl, whisk together the olive oil, lemon juice, salt, and pepper to make a dressing.
- Drizzle the dressing over the salad.
- Toss gently to combine.
- Serve immediately for a nutritious and quick lunch.

PALEO DIET

DINNER :

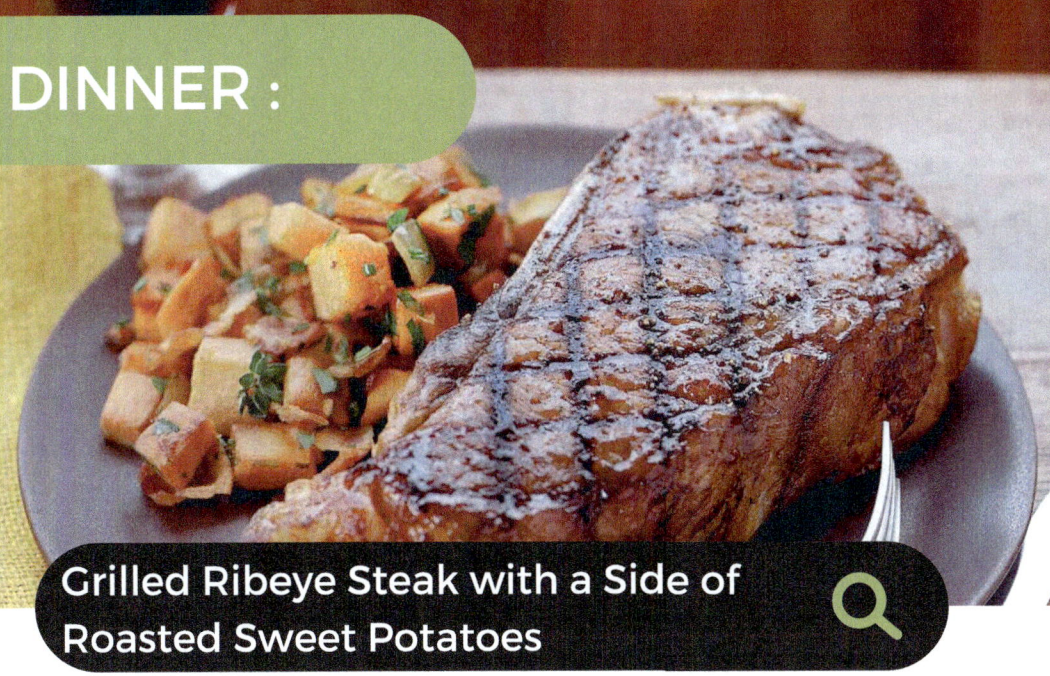

Grilled Ribeye Steak with a Side of Roasted Sweet Potatoes

INGREDIENTS

- 1 ribeye steak (about 6-8 oz)
- 1 medium sweet potato, peeled and cubed
- 1 tablespoon olive oil
- Salt and pepper, to taste
- 1/2 teaspoon garlic powder (optional)

PROCEDURE

- Preheat the oven to 400°F (200°C).
- Toss the sweet potato cubes with olive oil, salt, pepper, and garlic powder.
- Spread the sweet potatoes on a baking sheet and roast for 20-25 minutes, until tender and golden.
- Season the ribeye steak with salt and pepper.
- Grill the steak over medium-high heat to your preferred level of doneness, about 4-5 minutes per side for medium-rare.
- Let the steak rest for a few minutes before slicing.
- Serve the grilled steak alongside the roasted sweet potatoes.

BREAKFAST :

DAY14

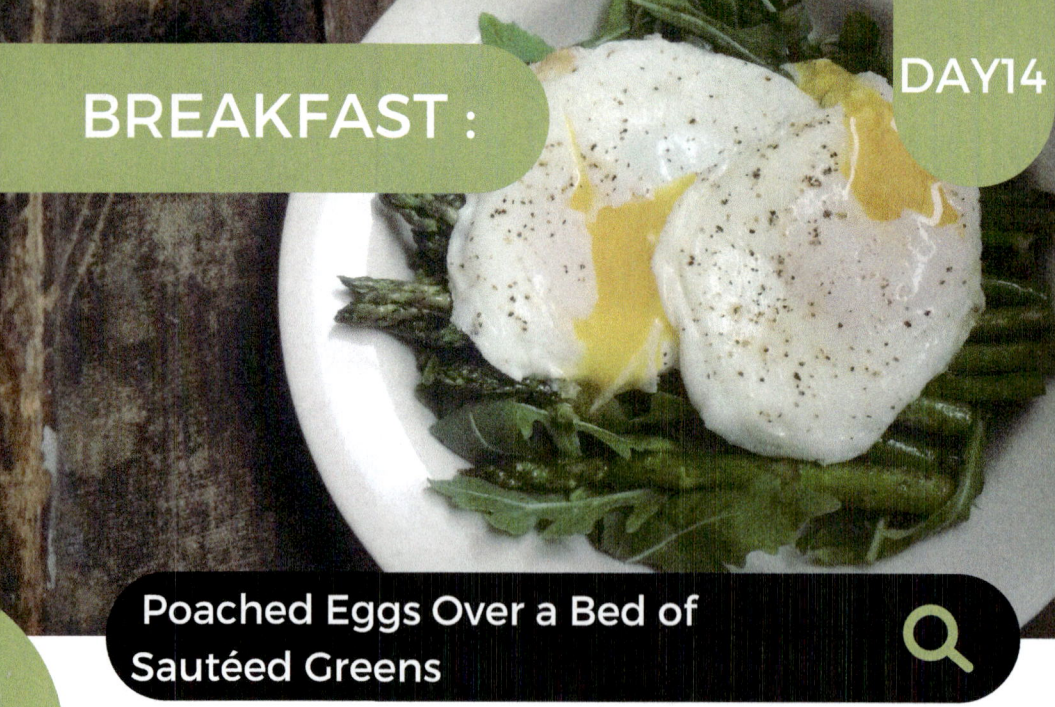

Poached Eggs Over a Bed of Sautéed Greens

INGREDIENTS

- 2 large eggs
- 2 cups mixed greens (like spinach, kale, or Swiss chard)
- 1 tablespoon olive oil
- Salt and pepper, to taste
- 1 teaspoon vinegar (for poaching eggs)

PROCEDURE

- Heat the olive oil in a skillet over medium heat.
- Add the mixed greens and sauté until wilted, about 2-3 minutes. Season with salt and pepper.
- To poach the eggs, bring a pot of water to a gentle simmer and add a teaspoon of vinegar.
- Crack each egg into a small bowl and gently slide them into the simmering water.
- Poach the eggs for about 3-4 minutes until the whites are set but yolks are still runny.
- Use a slotted spoon to remove the eggs from the water.
- Serve the poached eggs over the bed of sautéed greens.

PALEO DIET

LUNCH :

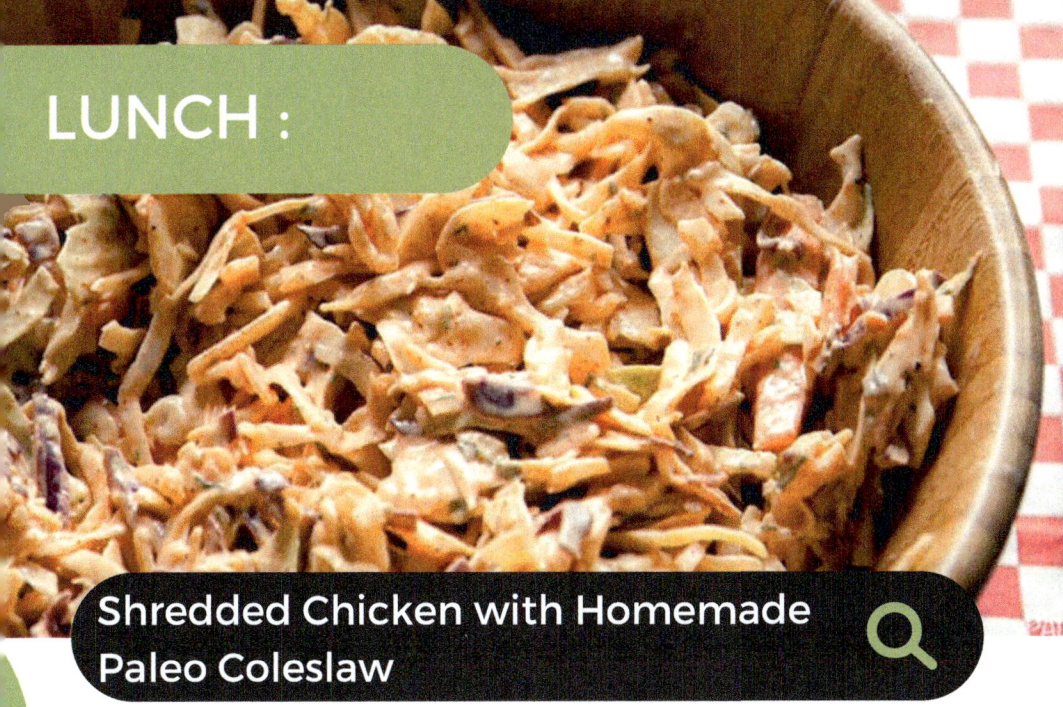

Shredded Chicken with Homemade Paleo Coleslaw

INGREDIENTS

- 1 cup shredded cabbage
- 1/2 carrot, shredded
- 1/4 cup Paleo-friendly mayonnaise
- 1 tablespoon apple cider vinegar
- Salt and pepper, to taste
- 1 small chicken breast, cooked and shredded

PROCEDURE

- In a bowl, combine the shredded cabbage and carrot.
- In a separate bowl, mix together the Paleo mayonnaise, apple cider vinegar, salt, and pepper to create a dressing.
- Toss the coleslaw with the dressing.
- Serve the coleslaw with the shredded chicken on top.

PALEO DIET

DINNER :

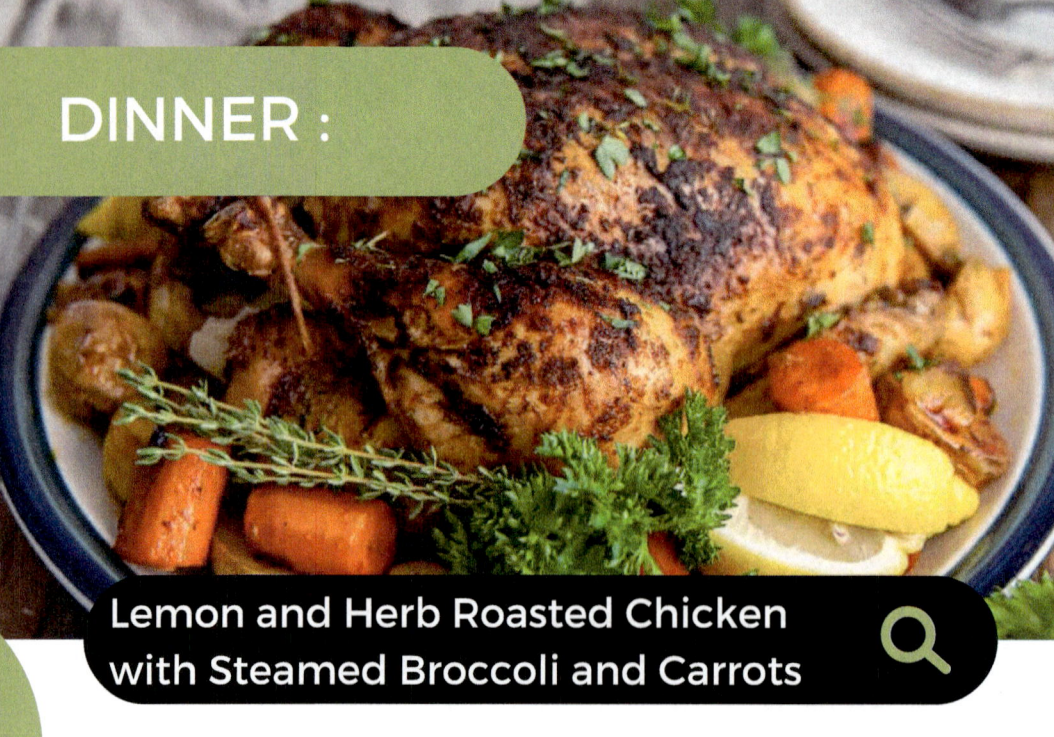

Lemon and Herb Roasted Chicken with Steamed Broccoli and Carrots

INGREDIENTS

- 1 small chicken breast
- 1/2 lemon, juiced and zested
- 1 tablespoon olive oil
- 1/2 teaspoon dried herbs (like thyme or rosemary)
- 1 cup broccoli florets
- 1/2 cup carrot slices
- Salt and pepper, to taste

PROCEDURE

- Preheat the oven to 375°F (190°C).
- In a bowl, mix together lemon juice and zest, olive oil, dried herbs, salt, and pepper.
- Coat the chicken breast with the lemon and herb mixture.
- Place the chicken in a baking dish and roast for about 25-30 minutes, or until fully cooked.
- Meanwhile, steam the broccoli and carrot slices until tender, about 5-7 minutes.
- Serve the lemon and herb roasted chicken with the steamed broccoli and carrots.

PALEO DIET

After completing Week 2, it's important to reflect on how your body has responded to the dietary changes. Use the following scale to rate your experiences in various aspects of your health and well-being. Rate each category from 1 to 10 (where 1 is 'no improvement' and 10 is 'significant improvement').

1. Digestive Comfort
- Question: How would you rate the overall comfort of your digestive system this week?
- Rating (1-10): _____

2. Energy Levels
- Question: How do you feel about your energy levels after following the meal plan for a week?
- Rating (1-10): _____

3. Sleep Quality
- Question: Have you noticed any changes in the quality of your sleep?
- Rating (1-10): _____

4. Mood and Mental Clarity
- Question: How has your mood and mental clarity been affected by the dietary changes?
- Rating (1-10): _____

5. Physical Comfort and Pain Levels
- Question: If you previously experienced any physical discomfort or pain, have you noticed any changes in its intensity or frequency?
- Rating (1-10): _____

6. Skin Health
- Question: Have there been any noticeable changes in your skin health/appearance?
- Rating (1-10): _____

7. Cravings and Appetite Control
- Question: How would you rate your control over cravings and appetite this week?
- Rating (1-10): _____

8. Overall Well-being
- Question: Considering all factors, how would you rate your overall well-being after Week 1?
- Rating (1-10): _____

WEEK 1

DIGESTIVE COMFORT	1	2	3	4	5	6	7	8	9	10
ENERGY LEVELS	1	2	3	4	5	6	7	8	9	10
SLEEP QUALITY	1	2	3	4	5	6	7	8	9	10
MOOD & MENTAL CLARITY	1	2	3	4	5	6	7	8	9	10
PHYSICAL COMFORT	1	2	3	4	5	6	7	8	9	10
SKIN HEALTH	1	2	3	4	5	6	7	8	9	10
CRAVINGS CONTROL	1	2	3	4	5	6	7	8	9	10
OVERALL WELL-BEING	1	2	3	4	5	6	7	8	9	10

notes

....
....
....
....
....
....
....
....

PALEO DIET

FOR SPECIAL *notes*

WEEK 3: EXPERIMENTING WITH FLAVORS

Week 3 is all about experimenting with flavors. It's time to get creative in the kitchen and try out new combinations of herbs, spices, and Paleo ingredients. This week challenges you to think outside the box and enjoy the process of cooking and tasting.

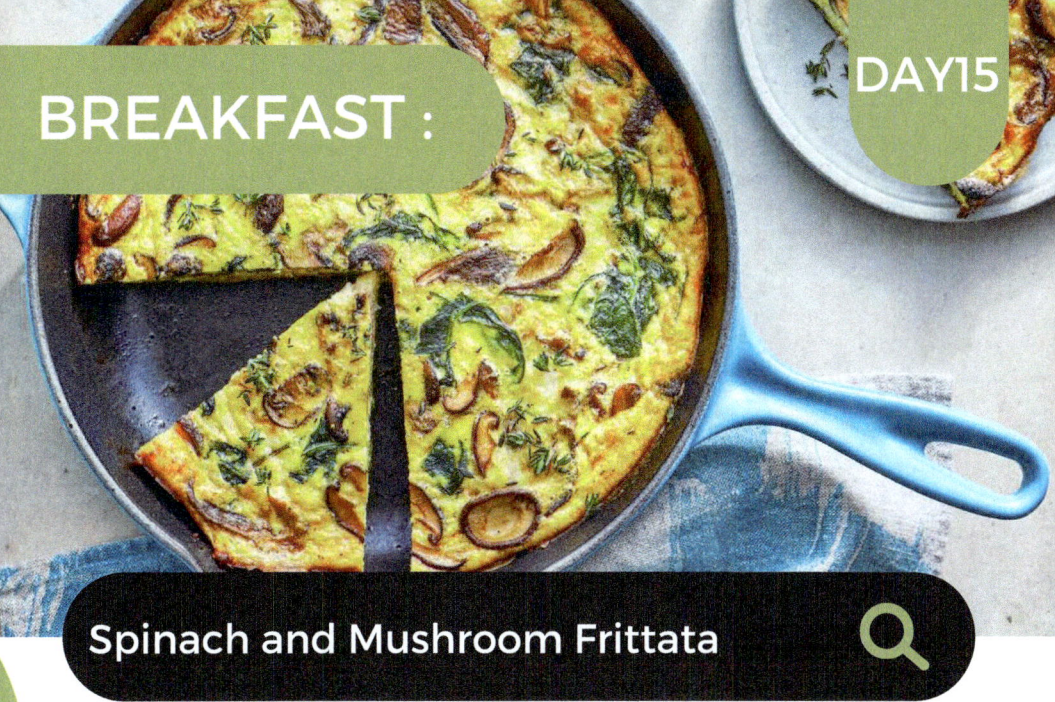

BREAKFAST :

DAY 15

Spinach and Mushroom Frittata

INGREDIENTS

- 2 large eggs
- 1 cup fresh spinach, chopped
- 1/2 cup mushrooms, sliced
- 1 tablespoon olive oil
- Salt and pepper, to taste

PROCEDURE

- Preheat the oven to 375°F (190°C).
- Heat the olive oil in an oven-safe skillet over medium heat.
- Add the mushrooms and sauté until they are soft, about 3-4 minutes.
- Add the spinach and cook until it wilts, about 1-2 minutes.
- Beat the eggs in a bowl, season with salt and pepper, and pour them over the vegetables.
- Cook without stirring for about 2 minutes until the edges start to set.
- Transfer the skillet to the oven and bake the frittata for 8-10 minutes, until the eggs are fully set.
- Serve the frittata warm.

PALEO DIET

LUNCH :

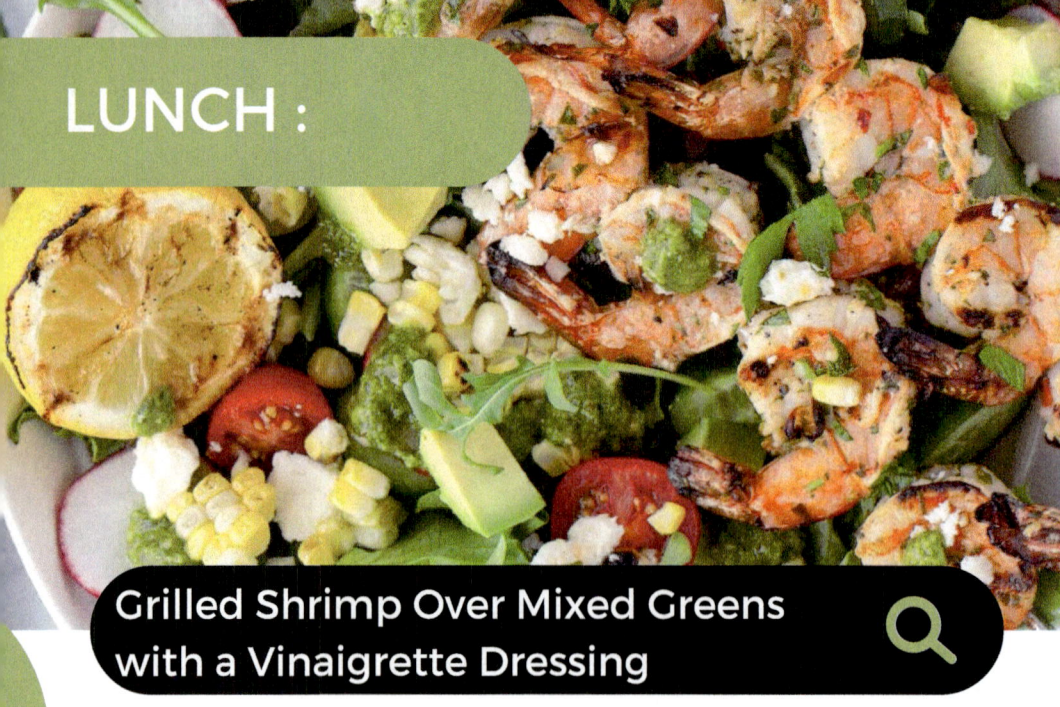

Grilled Shrimp Over Mixed Greens with a Vinaigrette Dressing

INGREDIENTS

- 5-6 large shrimp, peeled and deveined
- 2 cups mixed greens
- 2 tablespoons olive oil (divided)
- 1 tablespoon balsamic vinegar
- Salt and pepper, to taste

PROCEDURE

- Season the shrimp with salt and pepper.
- Heat 1 tablespoon of olive oil in a skillet over medium heat and grill the shrimp until pink and cooked through, about 2-3 minutes per side.
- In a bowl, whisk together the remaining olive oil and balsamic vinegar to make a dressing.
- Toss the mixed greens with the vinaigrette.
- Top the salad with the grilled shrimp.
- Serve immediately for a light and flavorful lunch.

DINNER :

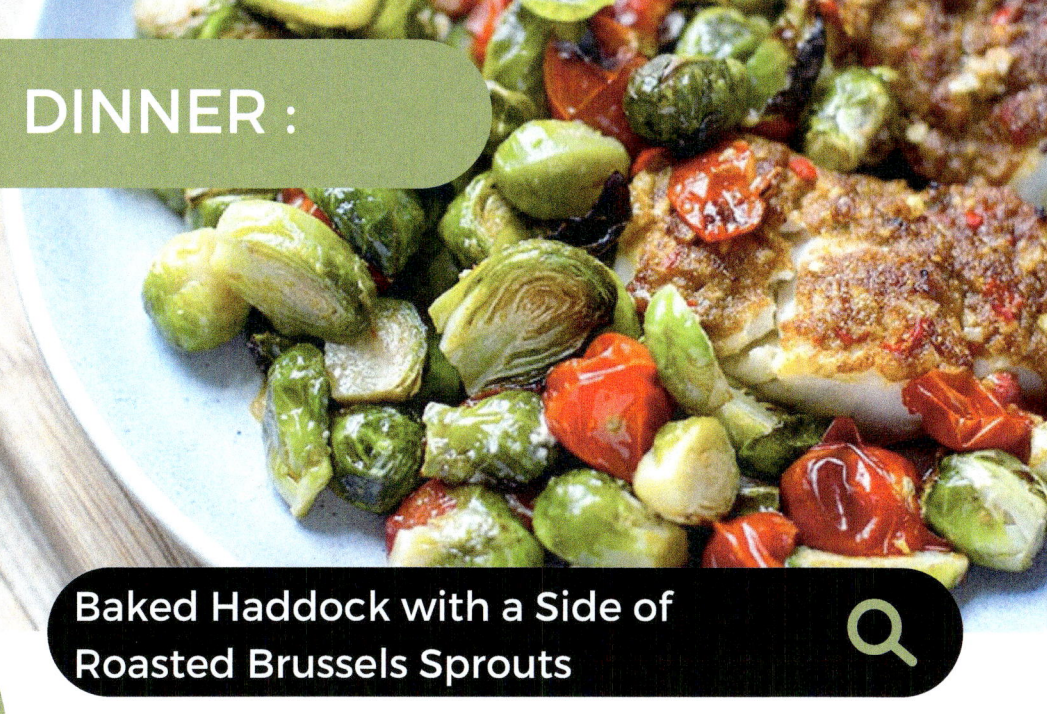

Baked Haddock with a Side of Roasted Brussels Sprouts

INGREDIENTS

- 1 haddock fillet (about 6 oz)
- 1 cup Brussels sprouts, halved
- 1 tablespoon olive oil
- Salt and pepper, to taste
- Lemon wedges, for serving

PROCEDURE

- Preheat the oven to 400°F (200°C).
- Toss the Brussels sprouts with half of the olive oil, salt, and pepper, and spread them on a baking sheet.
- Roast for 15-20 minutes, until tender and slightly browned.
- Season the haddock with salt, pepper, and the remaining olive oil.
- Place the haddock on a baking sheet lined with parchment paper.
- Bake for 12-15 minutes, or until the fish is cooked through and flakes easily.
- Serve the baked haddock with the roasted Brussels sprouts and a lemon wedge.

PALEO DIET

BREAKFAST :

DAY 16

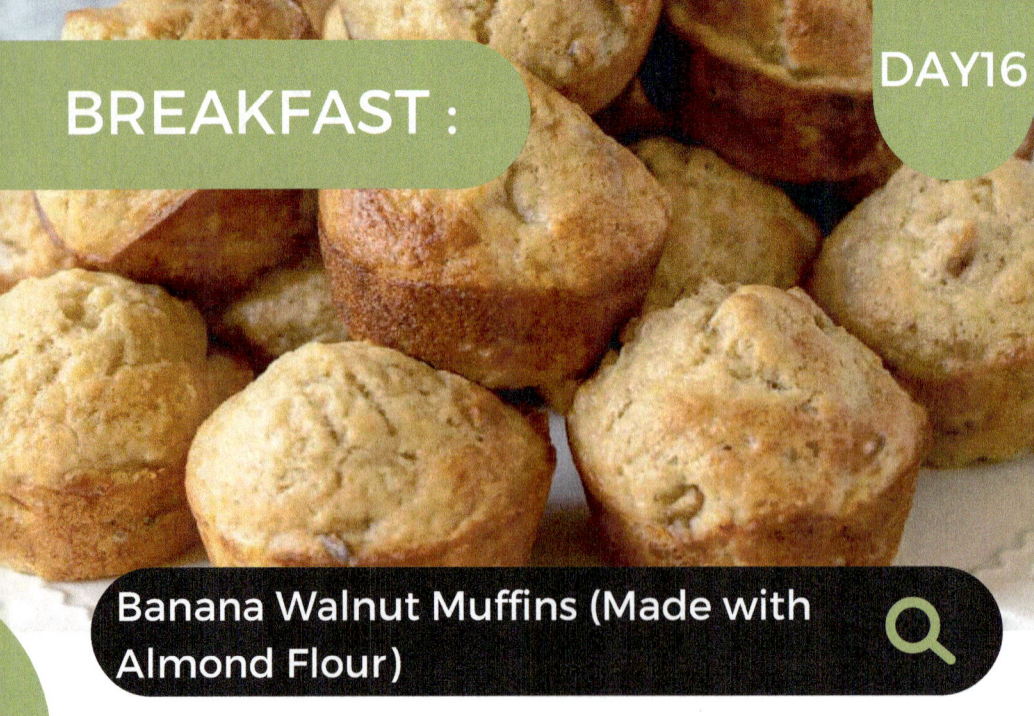

Banana Walnut Muffins (Made with Almond Flour)

INGREDIENTS

- 1 ripe banana, mashed
- 1 cup almond flour
- 2 large eggs
- 1/4 cup walnuts, chopped
- 1/4 teaspoon baking soda
- 1 tablespoon honey or maple syrup
- 1/2 teaspoon vanilla extract
- Pinch of salt

PROCEDURE

- Preheat the oven to 350°F (175°C) and line a muffin tin with paper liners.
- In a bowl, mix the mashed banana, eggs, honey, and vanilla extract.
- Add the almond flour, baking soda, and a pinch of salt to the wet ingredients. Stir until combined.
- Fold in the chopped walnuts.
- Divide the batter among the muffin cups.
- Bake for 15-20 minutes, or until a toothpick inserted into the center of a muffin comes out clean.
- Allow the muffins to cool before serving.

PALEO DIET

LUNCH :

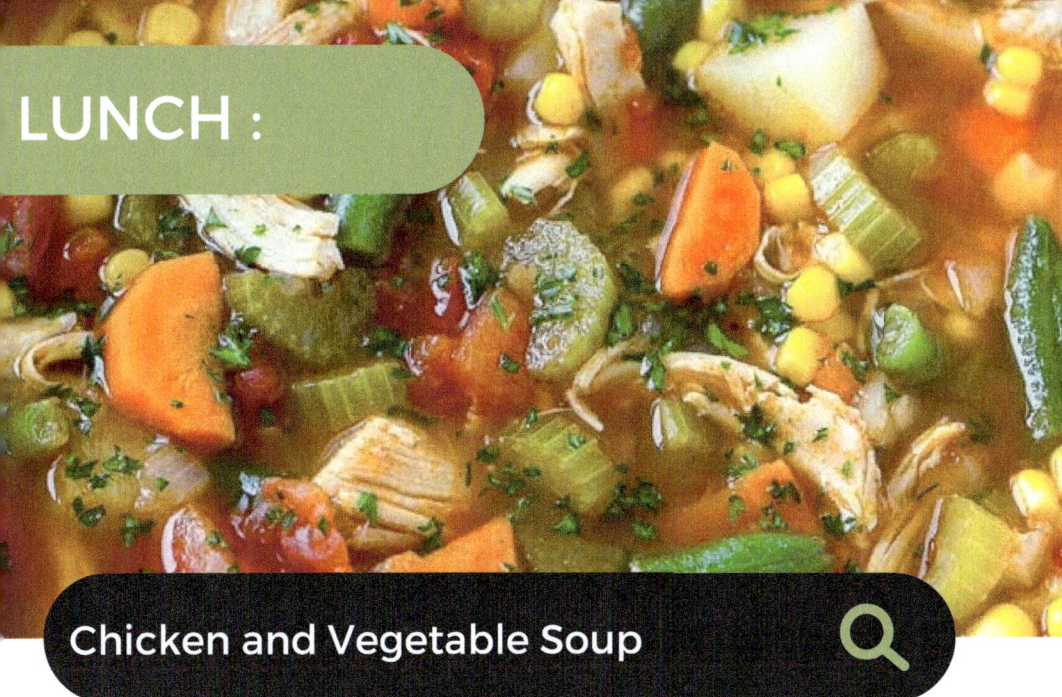

Chicken and Vegetable Soup

INGREDIENTS

- 1 small chicken breast, diced
- 1 cup mixed vegetables (carrots, celery, onions)
- 2 cups chicken broth (Paleo-friendly)
- 1 tablespoon olive oil
- Salt and pepper, to taste
- Fresh herbs (like parsley or thyme) for garnish

PROCEDURE

- Heat the olive oil in a pot over medium heat.
- Add the diced chicken and cook until browned.
- Add the mixed vegetables and sauté for a few minutes.
- Pour in the chicken broth and bring to a simmer.
- Season with salt and pepper.
- Simmer for about 15-20 minutes, until the vegetables are tender.
- Garnish with fresh herbs before serving.

PALEO DIET

DINNER :

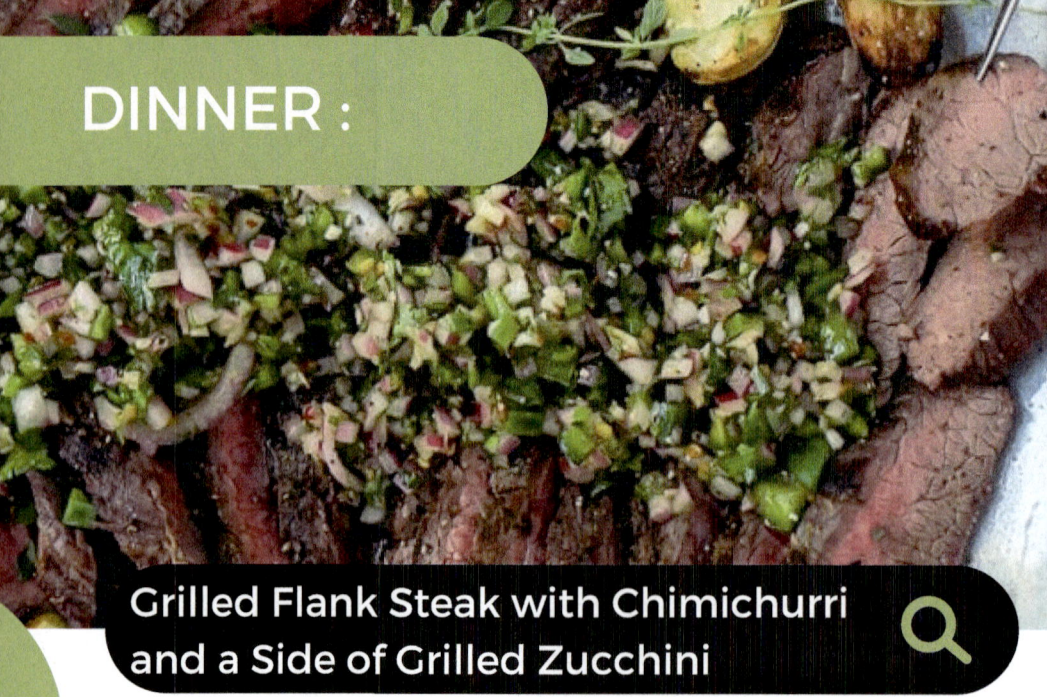

Grilled Flank Steak with Chimichurri and a Side of Grilled Zucchini

INGREDIENTS

- 1/2 cup fresh parsley, chopped
- 2 tablespoons olive oil
- 1 tablespoon red wine vinegar
- 1 garlic clove, minced
- Salt and red pepper flakes, to taste
- 1 flank steak (about 6-8 oz)
- 1 zucchini, sliced lengthwise
- Salt and pepper, to taste
- Olive oil for grilling

PROCEDURE

- For the chimichurri, mix together parsley, olive oil, red wine vinegar, garlic, salt, and red pepper flakes. Set aside.
- Season the flank steak and zucchini slices with salt and pepper.
- Brush the grill with olive oil and grill the steak over medium-high heat to your desired doneness, about 3-4 minutes per side for medium-rare.
- Grill the zucchini slices until tender and grill marks appear, about 2-3 minutes per side.
- Let the steak rest for a few minutes, then slice against the grain
- and serve with the grilled zucchini.
- Drizzle the chimichurri sauce over the sliced steak.
- Serve the grilled steak and zucchini with the fresh chimichurri sauce.

PALEO DIET

BREAKFAST :

DAY17

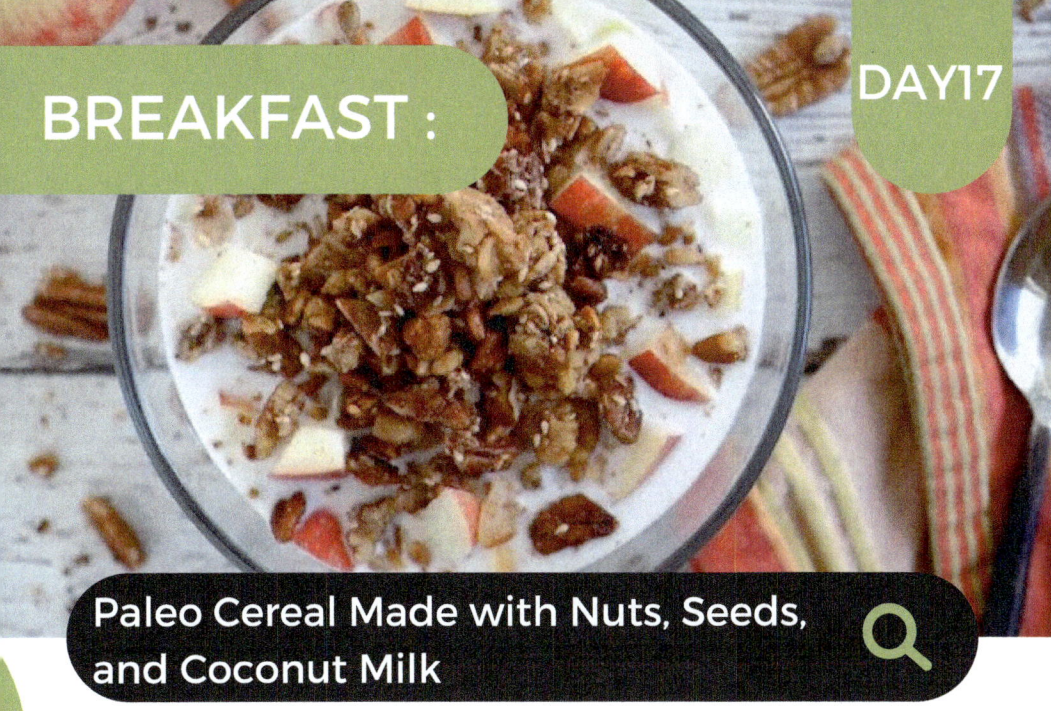

Paleo Cereal Made with Nuts, Seeds, and Coconut Milk

INGREDIENTS

- 1/4 cup mixed nuts (almonds, walnuts, pecans), roughly chopped
- 2 tablespoons pumpkin seeds
- 2 tablespoons shredded coconut (unsweetened)
- 1/2 teaspoon cinnamon
- 3/4 cup coconut milk (unsweetened)

PROCEDURE

- In a bowl, mix together the chopped nuts, pumpkin seeds, shredded coconut, and cinnamon.
- Pour the coconut milk over the nut and seed mixture.
- Stir well and let it sit for a few minutes to soften slightly.
- Serve as a nutritious Paleo-friendly cereal alternative.

PALEO DIET

LUNCH :

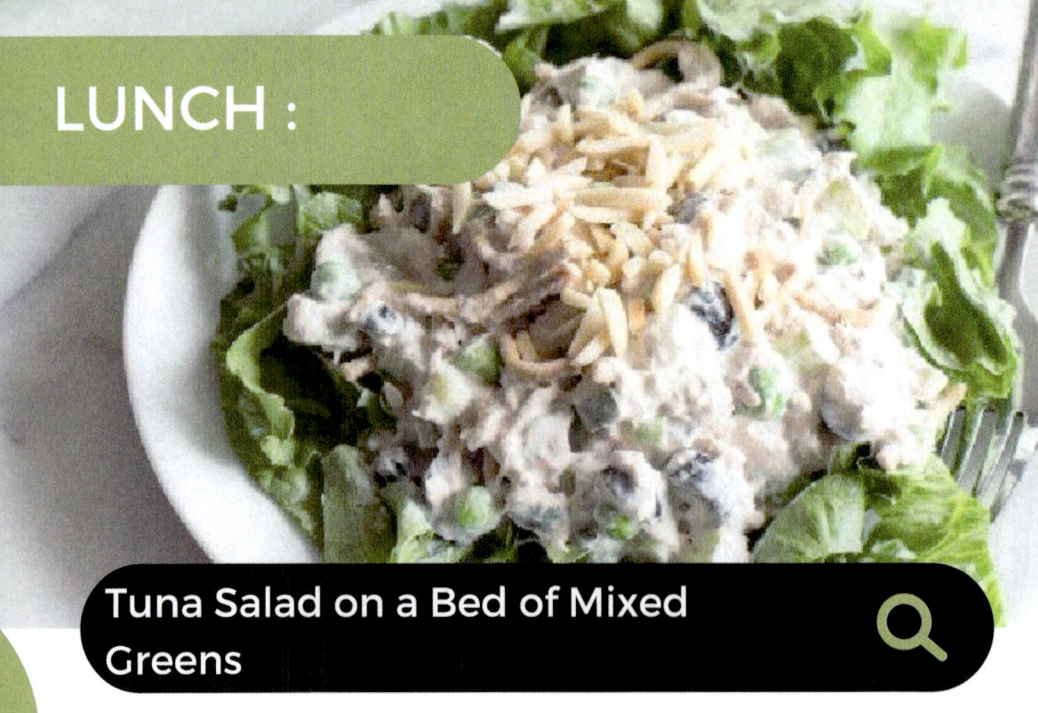

Tuna Salad on a Bed of Mixed Greens

INGREDIENTS

- 1 can of tuna in water, drained
- 2 cups mixed greens (like lettuce, arugula, spinach)
- 1/4 red onion, thinly sliced
- 2 tablespoons Paleo-friendly mayonnaise
- 1 teaspoon lemon juice
- Salt and pepper, to taste

PROCEDURE

- In a bowl, mix the tuna, mayonnaise, lemon juice, salt, and pepper.
- Place the mixed greens on a plate and top with the tuna mixture.
- Garnish with thinly sliced red onion.
- Serve immediately for a fresh and satisfying lunch.

DINNER :

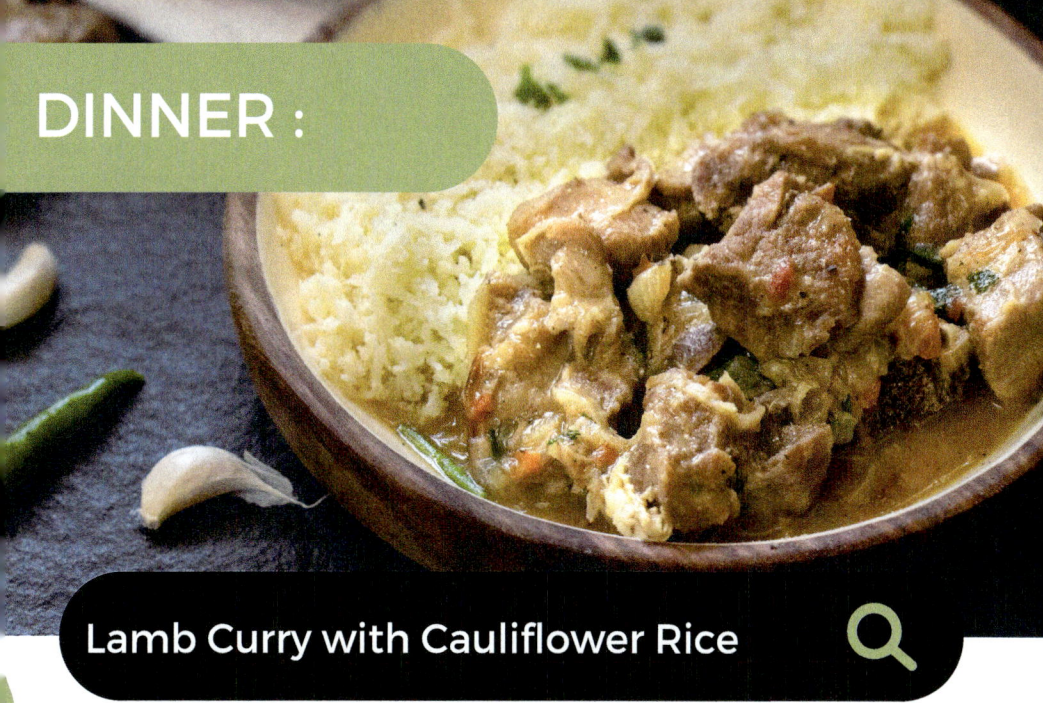

Lamb Curry with Cauliflower Rice

INGREDIENTS

- 1/2 lb lamb, cut into cubes
- 1/2 onion, finely chopped
- 1 garlic clove, minced
- 1 tablespoon curry powder
- 1/2 can coconut milk
- 1 tablespoon olive oil
- Salt and pepper, to taste

Ingredients for Cauliflower Rice:
- 1/2 head cauliflower, grated or processed into rice-sized pieces
- 1 tablespoon olive oil
- Salt, to taste

PROCEDURE

- Heat olive oil in a pan over medium heat. Add the onion and garlic, sautéing until soft.
- Add the lamb cubes, browning them on all sides.
- Stir in the curry powder, then pour in the coconut milk. Bring to a simmer.
- Reduce heat and simmer for about 20 minutes, until the lamb is tender.
- For the cauliflower rice, heat olive oil in a separate pan. Add the grated cauliflower and sauté for 5-7 minutes until tender. Season with salt.
- Serve the lamb curry over the cauliflower rice.

PALEO DIET

BREAKFAST :

DAY18

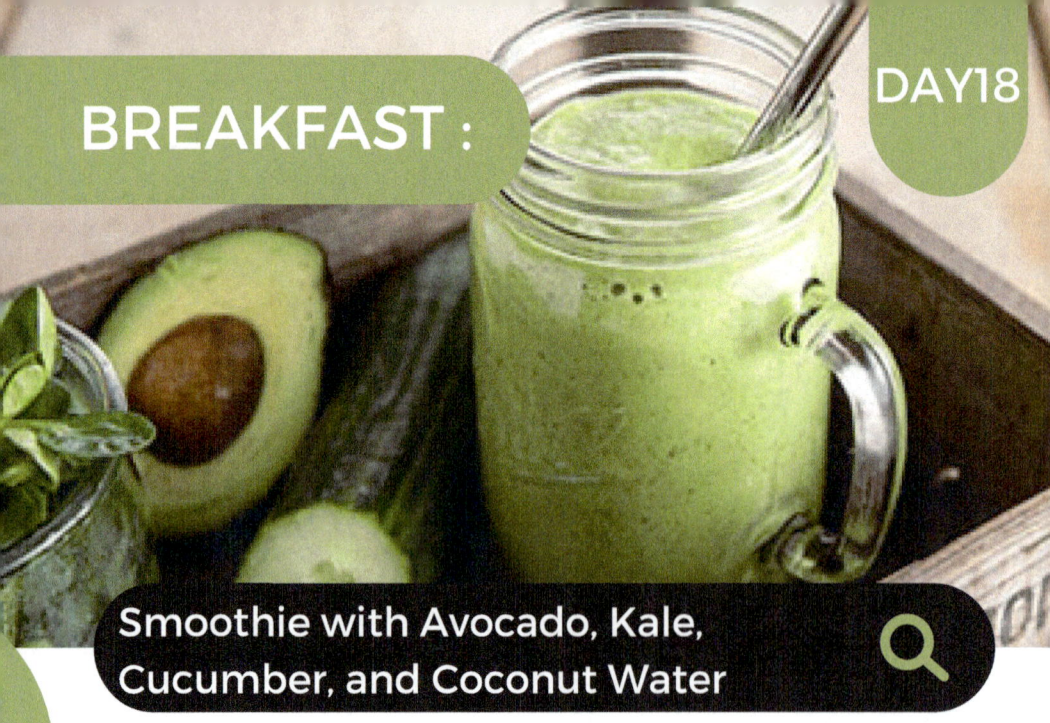

Smoothie with Avocado, Kale, Cucumber, and Coconut Water

INGREDIENTS

- 1/2 ripe avocado
- 1 cup kale, stems removed
- 1/2 cucumber, peeled and sliced
- 1 cup coconut water
- Ice cubes (optional)

PROCEDURE

- Combine the avocado, kale, cucumber, and coconut water in a blender.
- Add ice cubes if desired for a colder smoothie.
- Blend until smooth and creamy.
- Serve immediately in a tall glass for a nutrient-rich start to your day.

PALEO DIET

LUNCH :

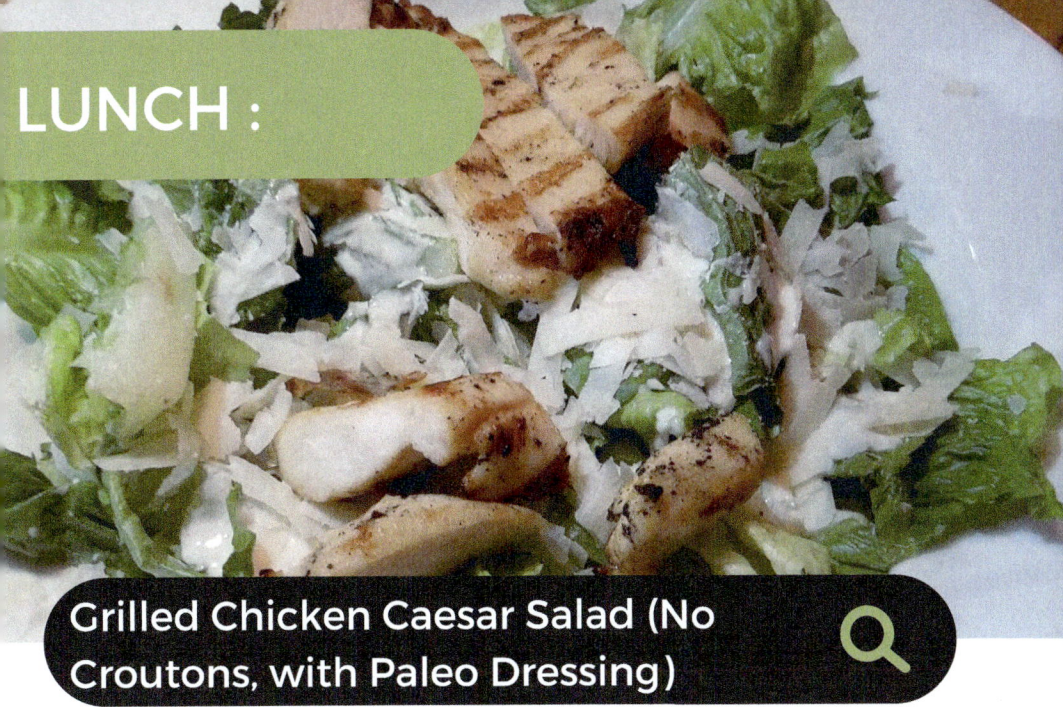

Grilled Chicken Caesar Salad (No Croutons, with Paleo Dressing)

INGREDIENTS

- 1 small chicken breast, grilled and sliced
- 2 cups Romaine lettuce, chopped
- Paleo-friendly Caesar dressing (homemade or store-bought)
- 1 tablespoon grated Parmesan cheese (optional, omit for strict Paleo)

PROCEDURE

- Place the chopped Romaine lettuce in a large bowl.
- Top with the sliced grilled chicken.
- Drizzle with Paleo-friendly Caesar dressing.
- Optionally, sprinkle with Parmesan cheese if included in your diet.
- Toss the salad lightly and serve.

PALEO DIET

DINNER :

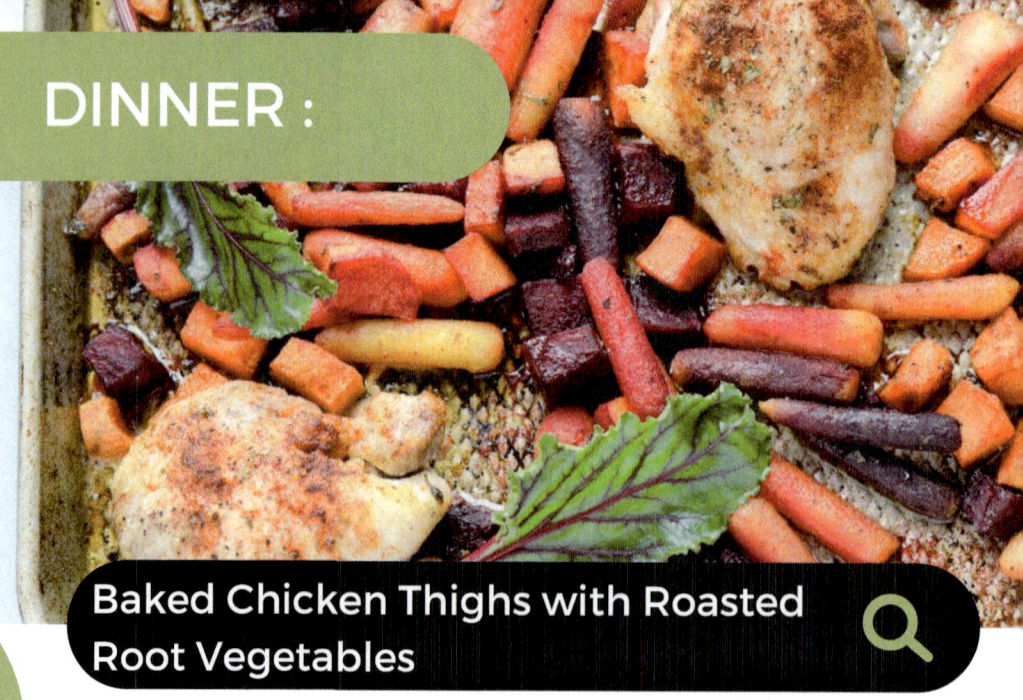

Baked Chicken Thighs with Roasted Root Vegetables

INGREDIENTS

- 2 chicken thighs, bone-in and skin-on
- 1 cup mixed root vegetables (carrots, parsnips, turnips), peeled and diced
- 2 tablespoons olive oil
- Salt and pepper, to taste
- Herbs (like thyme or rosemary), for seasoning

PROCEDURE

- Preheat the oven to 400°F (200°C).
- Toss the diced root vegetables with 1 tablespoon of olive oil, salt, pepper, and herbs. Spread them in a single layer on a baking sheet.
- Rub the chicken thighs with the remaining olive oil, salt, pepper, and additional herbs.
- Place the chicken thighs on the baking sheet with the vegetables.
- Bake for about 35-40 minutes, until the chicken is cooked through and the vegetables are tender.
- Serve the chicken thighs with the roasted root vegetables.

PALEO DIET

BREAKFAST :

DAY19

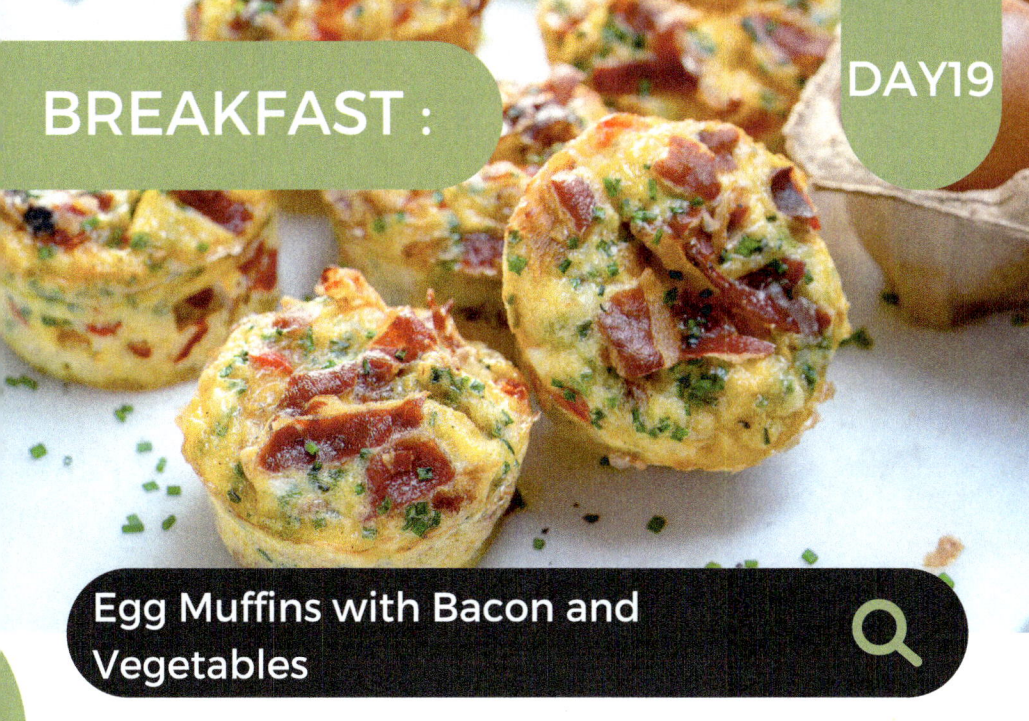

Egg Muffins with Bacon and Vegetables

INGREDIENTS

- 4 large eggs
- 2 slices of bacon, cooked and crumbled
- 1/4 cup bell pepper, diced
- 1/4 cup spinach, chopped
- Salt and pepper, to taste
- Cooking spray or olive oil (for greasing muffin tin)

PROCEDURE

- Preheat the oven to 350°F (175°C) and grease a muffin tin with cooking spray or olive oil.
- In a bowl, whisk the eggs and season with salt and pepper.
- Stir in the crumbled bacon, diced bell pepper, and chopped spinach.
- Pour the mixture into the muffin tin, filling each cup about 2/3 full.
- Bake for 15-20 minutes, or until the egg muffins are set and lightly golden on top.
- Let them cool for a few minutes before removing from the tin.
- Serve the egg muffins warm.

PALEO DIET

LUNCH :

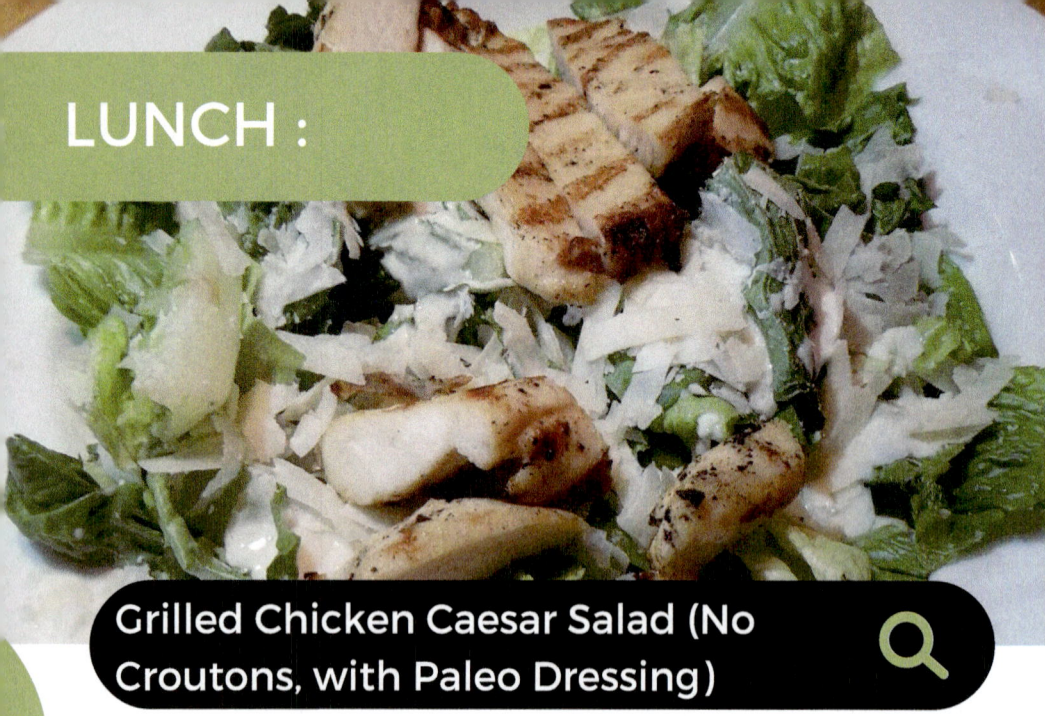

Grilled Chicken Caesar Salad (No Croutons, with Paleo Dressing)

INGREDIENTS

- 1 small chicken breast, grilled and sliced
- 2 cups Romaine lettuce, chopped
- Paleo-friendly Caesar dressing (homemade or store-bought)
- 1 tablespoon grated Parmesan cheese (optional, omit for strict Paleo)

PROCEDURE

- Place the chopped Romaine lettuce in a large bowl.
- Top with the sliced grilled chicken.
- Drizzle with Paleo-friendly Caesar dressing.
- Optionally, sprinkle with Parmesan cheese if included in your diet.
- Toss the salad lightly and serve.

DINNER :

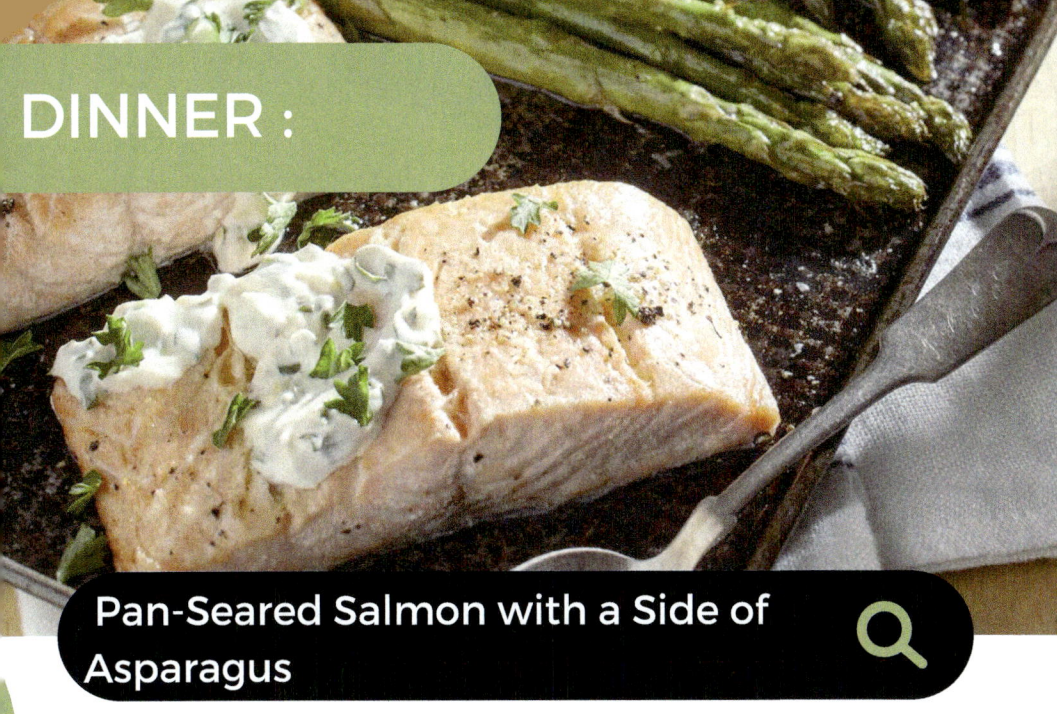

Pan-Seared Salmon with a Side of Asparagus

INGREDIENTS

- 1 salmon fillet (about 6 oz)
- 1 cup asparagus spears, ends trimmed
- 1 tablespoon olive oil
- Salt and pepper, to taste
- Lemon wedges, for serving

PROCEDURE

- Season the salmon with salt and pepper.
- Heat the olive oil in a skillet over medium-high heat.
- Place the salmon in the skillet, skin-side down, and cook for about 4-5 minutes.
- Flip the salmon and cook for another 3-4 minutes, or until it's cooked to your liking.
- In another skillet or in the same skillet, sauté the asparagus with a bit of olive oil, salt, and pepper until tender-crisp, about 4-5 minutes.
- Serve the pan-seared salmon with the sautéed asparagus and a lemon wedge on the side.

PALEO DIET

BREAKFAST :

DAY 20

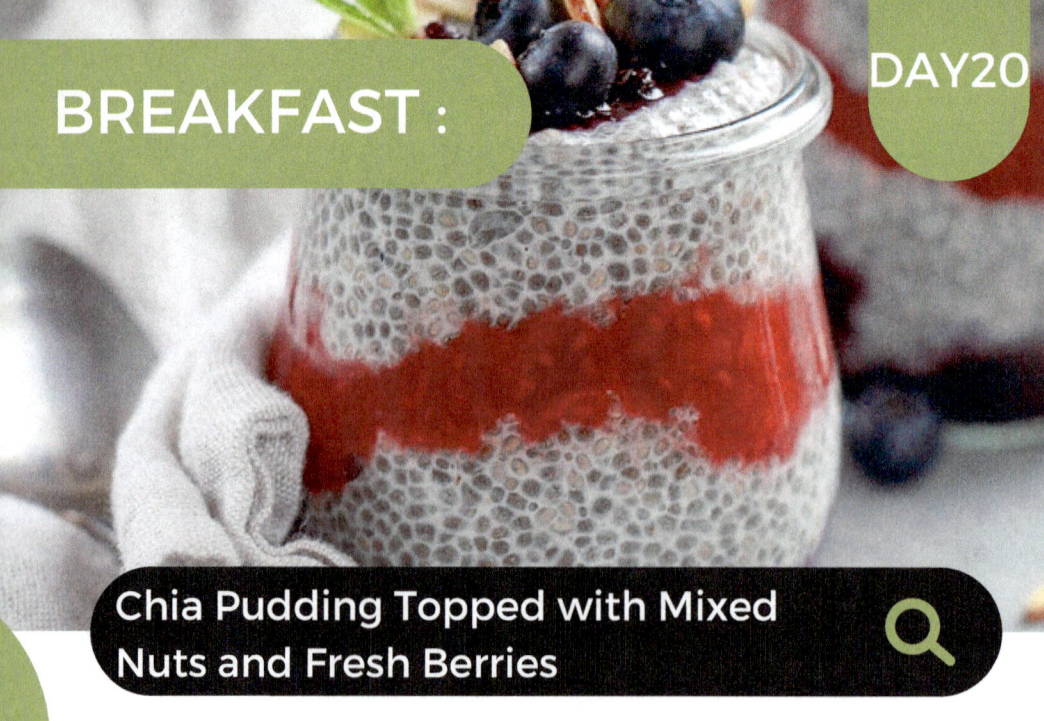

Chia Pudding Topped with Mixed Nuts and Fresh Berries

INGREDIENTS

- 3 tablespoons chia seeds
- 3/4 cup coconut milk (unsweetened)
- 1/4 teaspoon vanilla extract (optional)
- 1 tablespoon honey or maple syrup (optional)
- 1/4 cup mixed nuts (almonds, walnuts, pecans), roughly chopped
- 1/2 cup fresh berries (strawberries, blueberries, raspberries)

PROCEDURE

- In a bowl, mix the chia seeds with coconut milk, vanilla extract (if using), and honey or maple syrup (if using).
- Stir well to combine and let sit for 5 minutes, then stir again to prevent clumping.
- Cover and refrigerate for at least 2 hours, preferably overnight, until it achieves a pudding-like consistency.
- Top the chia pudding with chopped mixed nuts and fresh berries before serving.

PALEO DIET

LUNCH :

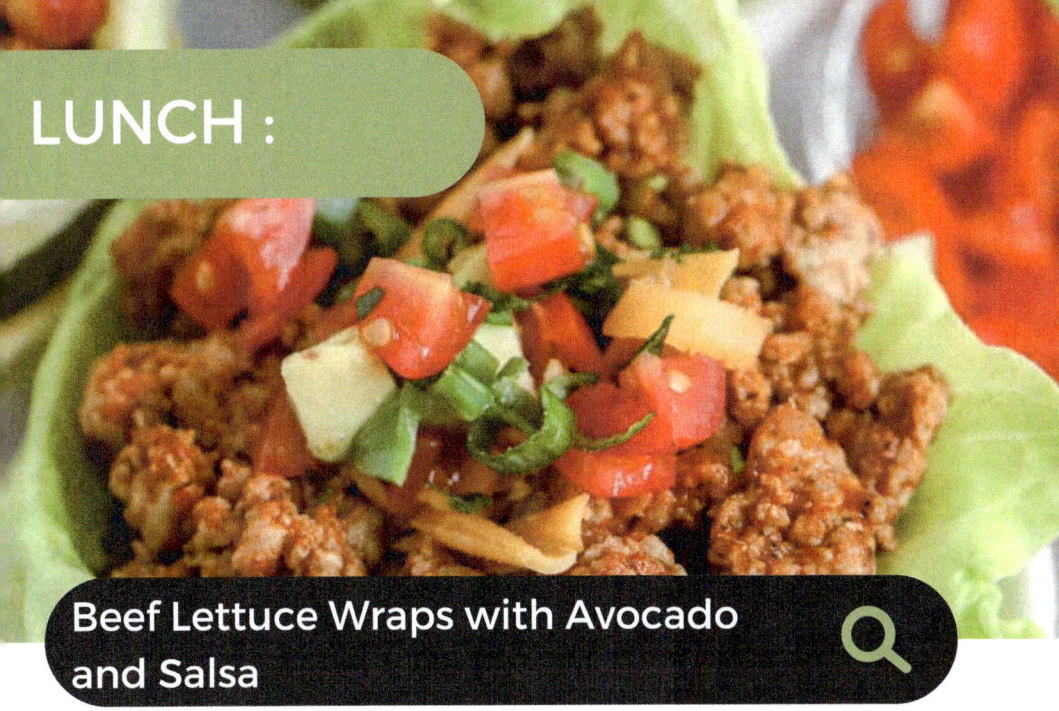

Beef Lettuce Wraps with Avocado and Salsa

INGREDIENTS

- 1/2 lb beef (flank steak or ground beef), cooked and sliced or crumbled
- 4-5 large lettuce leaves (such as Romaine or Butter lettuce)
- 1/2 ripe avocado, diced
- Salsa (ensure it's Paleo-friendly)
- Salt and pepper, to taste

PROCEDURE

- Season the cooked beef with salt and pepper.
- Place a spoonful of beef on each lettuce leaf.
- Top the beef with diced avocado and a spoonful of salsa.
- Roll up the lettuce leaves to enclose the filling.
- Serve immediately for a flavorful and light lunch.

DINNER :

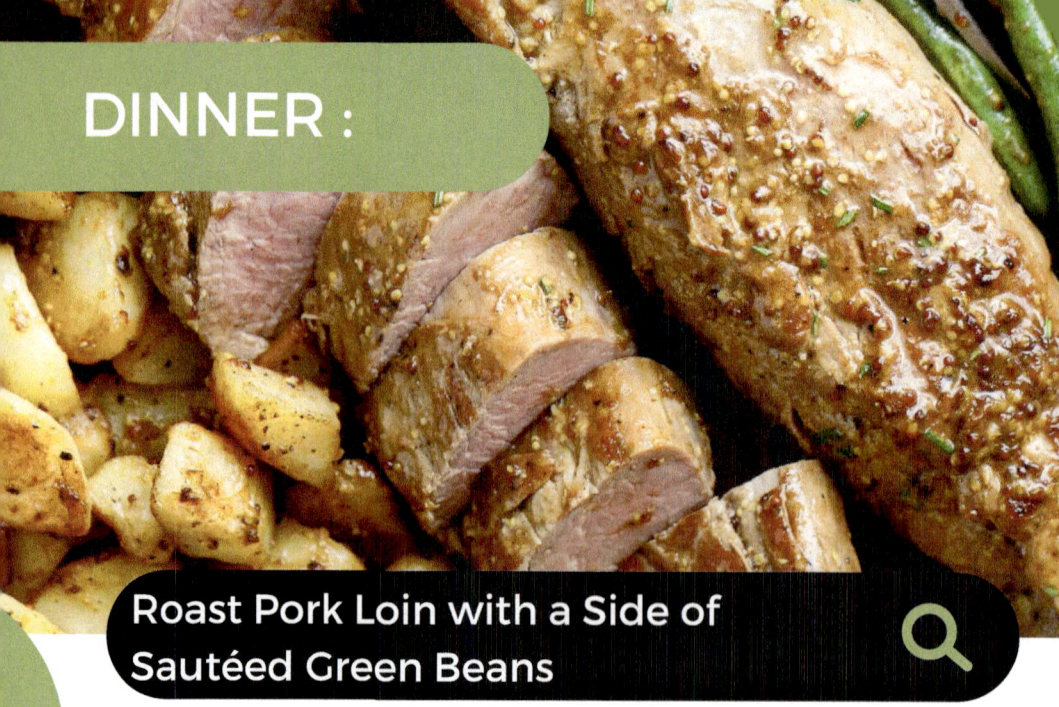

Roast Pork Loin with a Side of Sautéed Green Beans

INGREDIENTS

- 1 pork loin (about 6-8 oz)
- Salt and pepper, to taste
- 1 cup green beans, ends trimmed
- 1 tablespoon olive oil
- 1 garlic clove, minced

PROCEDURE

- Preheat the oven to 375°F (190°C).
- Season the pork loin with salt and pepper.
- Place the pork loin in a roasting pan and roast in the oven for about 20-25 minutes, or until it reaches an internal temperature of 145°F (63°C).
- While the pork is roasting, heat olive oil in a skillet over medium heat.
- Add minced garlic and green beans, sautéing until the beans are tender and slightly browned, about 5-7 minutes.
- Season the green beans with salt and pepper.
- Serve the roast pork loin with the sautéed green beans on the side.

PALEO DIET

BREAKFAST :

DAY 21

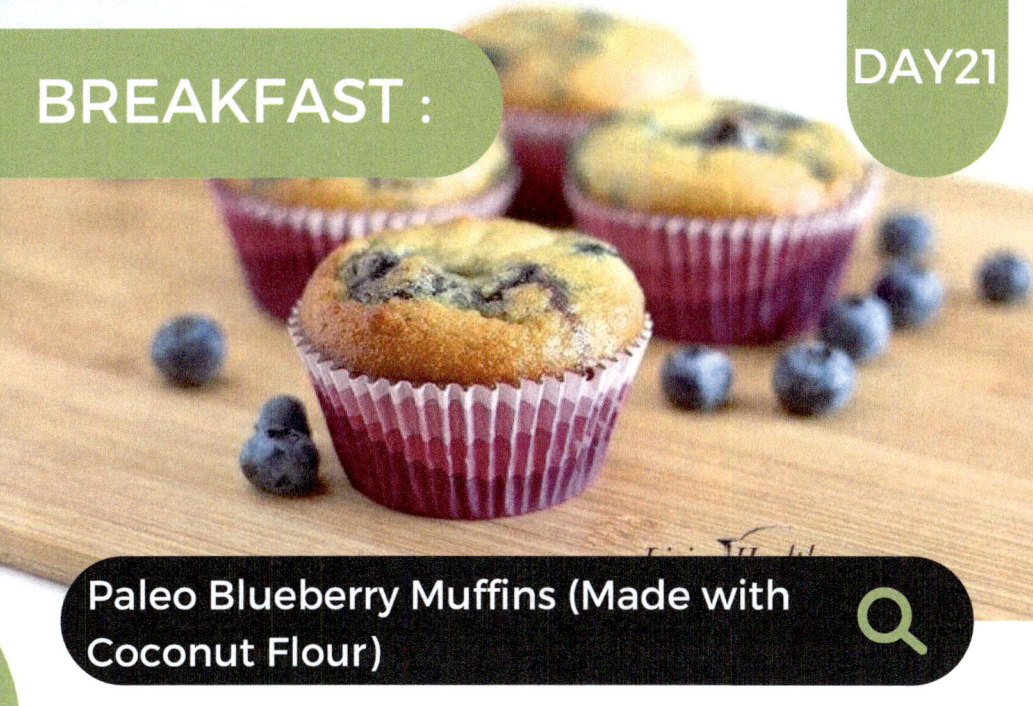

Paleo Blueberry Muffins (Made with Coconut Flour)

INGREDIENTS

- 1/2 cup coconut flour
- 1/4 cup honey or maple syrup
- 4 large eggs
- 1/4 cup coconut oil, melted
- 1/2 teaspoon baking powder
- 1/2 teaspoon vanilla extract
- 1/2 cup fresh blueberries
- Pinch of salt

PROCEDURE

- Preheat the oven to 350°F (175°C) and line a muffin tin with paper liners.
- In a bowl, mix together the coconut flour, baking powder, and salt.
- In another bowl, whisk the eggs, honey or maple syrup, melted coconut oil, and vanilla extract.
- Combine the wet and dry ingredients until smooth.
- Gently fold in the blueberries.
- Divide the batter among the muffin cups.
- Bake for 18-22 minutes, or until a toothpick inserted into the center comes out clean.
- Let the muffins cool before serving.

PALEO DIET

LUNCH :

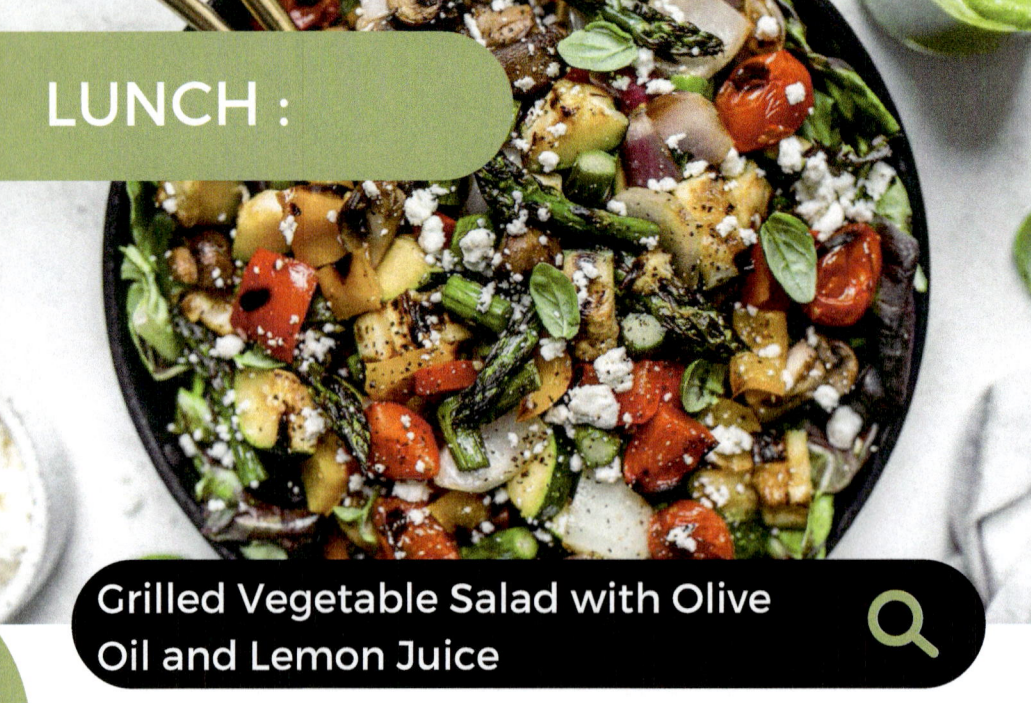

Grilled Vegetable Salad with Olive Oil and Lemon Juice

INGREDIENTS

- 1 bell pepper, sliced
- 1 zucchini, sliced
- 1/2 red onion, sliced
- 2 cups mixed greens
- 2 tablespoons olive oil (plus more for grilling)
- 1 tablespoon lemon juice
- Salt and pepper, to taste

PROCEDURE

- Toss the bell pepper, zucchini, and red onion with a little olive oil, salt, and pepper.
- Grill the vegetables over medium heat until tender and slightly charred.
- In a large bowl, combine the grilled vegetables with the mixed greens.
- Whisk together 2 tablespoons of olive oil and lemon juice, and season with salt and pepper.
- Drizzle the dressing over the salad and toss to combine.
- Serve the grilled vegetable salad for a light and refreshing lunch.

PALEO DIET

DINNER :

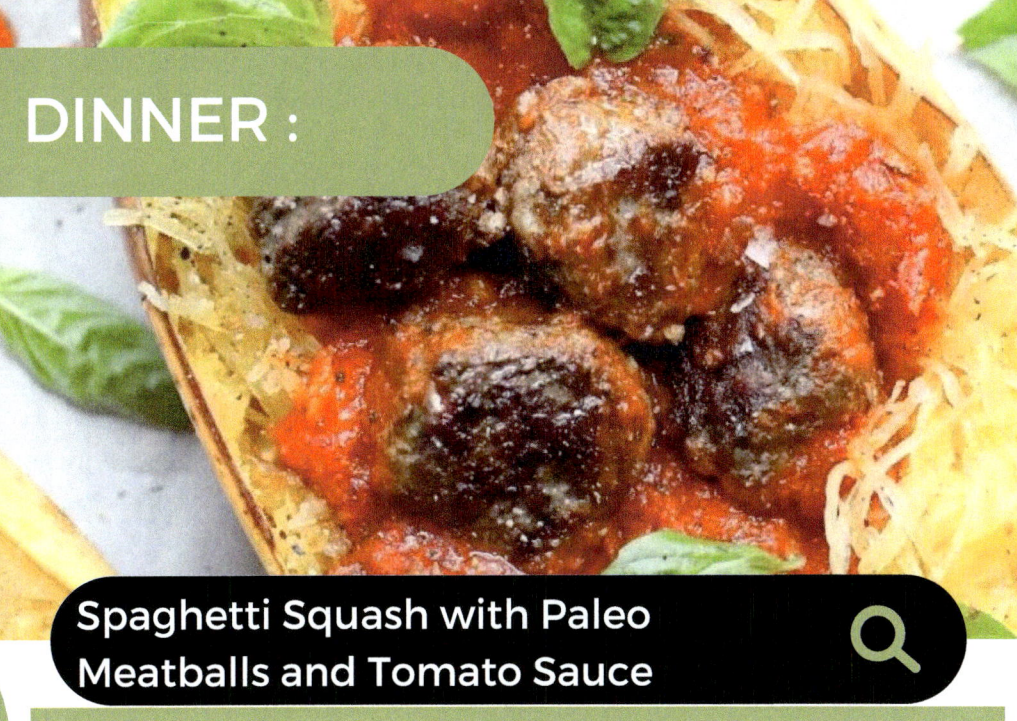

Spaghetti Squash with Paleo Meatballs and Tomato Sauce

INGREDIENTS

- 1/2 lb ground beef or turkey
- 1/4 onion, finely chopped
- 1 garlic clove, minced
- 1/2 teaspoon Italian seasoning
- Salt and pepper, to taste

Ingredients for Spaghetti Squash and Sauce:
- 1 small spaghetti squash
- 1 cup Paleo-friendly tomato sauce
- Olive oil
- Salt and pepper, to taste

PROCEDURE

- Preheat the oven to 400°F (200°C).
- Cut the spaghetti squash in half lengthwise and remove the seeds. Season with olive oil, salt, and pepper.
- Place the squash cut-side down on a baking sheet and roast for 30-40 minutes, until tender.
- For the meatballs, combine the ground meat, onion, garlic, Italian seasoning, salt, and pepper. Form into small balls.
- Bake the meatballs in the oven for 20-25 minutes, or until cooked through.
- Heat the tomato sauce in a saucepan.
- Use a fork to scrape the spaghetti squash into strands.
- Serve the spaghetti squash topped with meatballs and tomato sauce.

PALEO DIET

After completing Week 3, it's important to reflect on how your body has responded to the dietary changes. Use the following scale to rate your experiences in various aspects of your health and well-being. Rate each category from 1 to 10 (where 1 is 'no improvement' and 10 is 'significant improvement').

1. Digestive Comfort
- Question: How would you rate the overall comfort of your digestive system this week?
- Rating (1-10): _____

2. Energy Levels
- Question: How do you feel about your energy levels after following the meal plan for a week?
- Rating (1-10): _____

3. Sleep Quality
- Question: Have you noticed any changes in the quality of your sleep?
- Rating (1-10): _____

4. Mood and Mental Clarity
- Question: How has your mood and mental clarity been affected by the dietary changes?
- Rating (1-10): _____

5. Physical Comfort and Pain Levels
- Question: If you previously experienced any physical discomfort or pain, have you noticed any changes in its intensity or frequency?
- Rating (1-10): _____

6. Skin Health
- Question: Have there been any noticeable changes in your skin health/appearance?
- Rating (1-10): _____

7. Cravings and Appetite Control
- Question: How would you rate your control over cravings and appetite this week?
- Rating (1-10): _____

8. Overall Well-being
- Question: Considering all factors, how would you rate your overall well-being after Week 1?
- Rating (1-10): _____

WEEK 1

DIGESTIVE COMFORT	1	2	3	4	5	6	7	8	9	10
ENERGY LEVELS	1	2	3	4	5	6	7	8	9	10
SLEEP QUALITY	1	2	3	4	5	6	7	8	9	10
MOOD & MENTAL CLARITY	1	2	3	4	5	6	7	8	9	10
PHYSICAL COMFORT	1	2	3	4	5	6	7	8	9	10
SKIN HEALTH	1	2	3	4	5	6	7	8	9	10
CRAVINGS CONTROL	1	2	3	4	5	6	7	8	9	10
OVERALL WELL-BEING	1	2	3	4	5	6	7	8	9	10

notes

PALEO DIET

FOR SPECIAL *notes*

WEEK 4: REFINING YOUR FAVORITES

Welcome to the final week of your Paleo meal plan. This week is about refining your favorites. Revisit the meals you loved most and feel free to repeat them. It's also a good time to tweak and perfect any recipes to suit your taste.

BREAKFAST :

DAY22

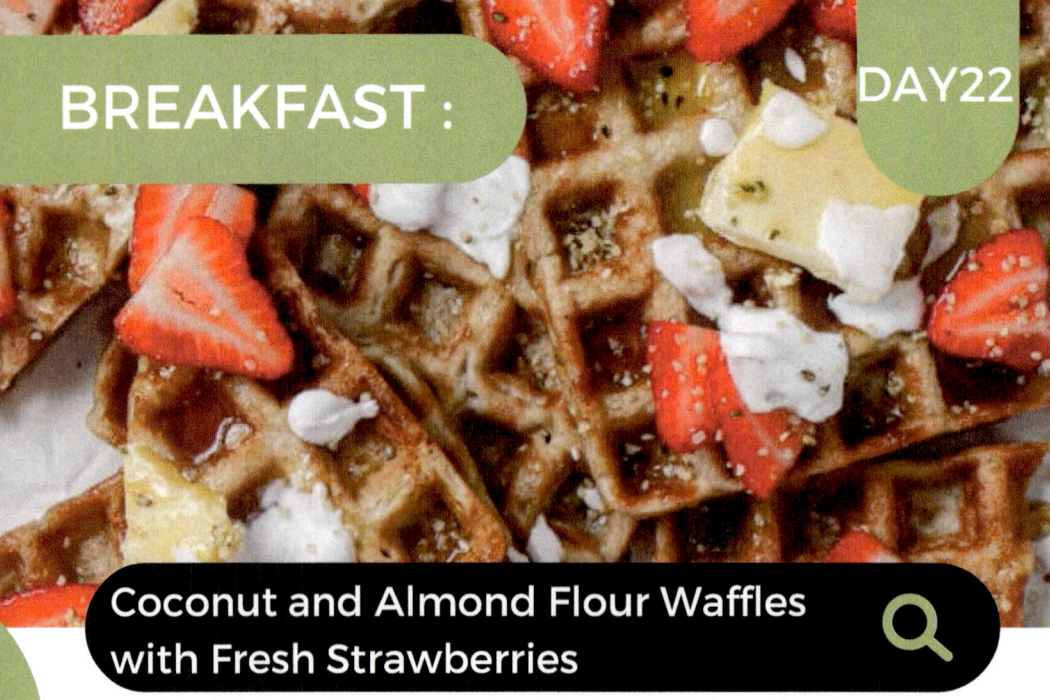

Coconut and Almond Flour Waffles with Fresh Strawberries

INGREDIENTS

- 1/2 cup almond flour
- 1/4 cup coconut flour
- 2 large eggs
- 1/2 cup almond milk (unsweetened)
- 1 tablespoon honey or maple syrup
- 1 teaspoon baking powder
- 1/2 teaspoon vanilla extract
- Pinch of salt
- Cooking spray or coconut oil (for waffle iron)
- Fresh strawberries for topping

PROCEDURE

- Preheat your waffle iron.
- In a bowl, mix together the almond flour, coconut flour, baking powder, and a pinch of salt.
- In another bowl, whisk the eggs, almond milk, honey or maple syrup, and vanilla extract.
- Combine the wet and dry ingredients, stirring until smooth.
- Grease the waffle iron with cooking spray or coconut oil.
- Pour the batter onto the waffle iron and cook according to the manufacturer's instructions, until golden brown.
- Serve the waffles topped with fresh strawberries.

PALEO DIET

LUNCH :

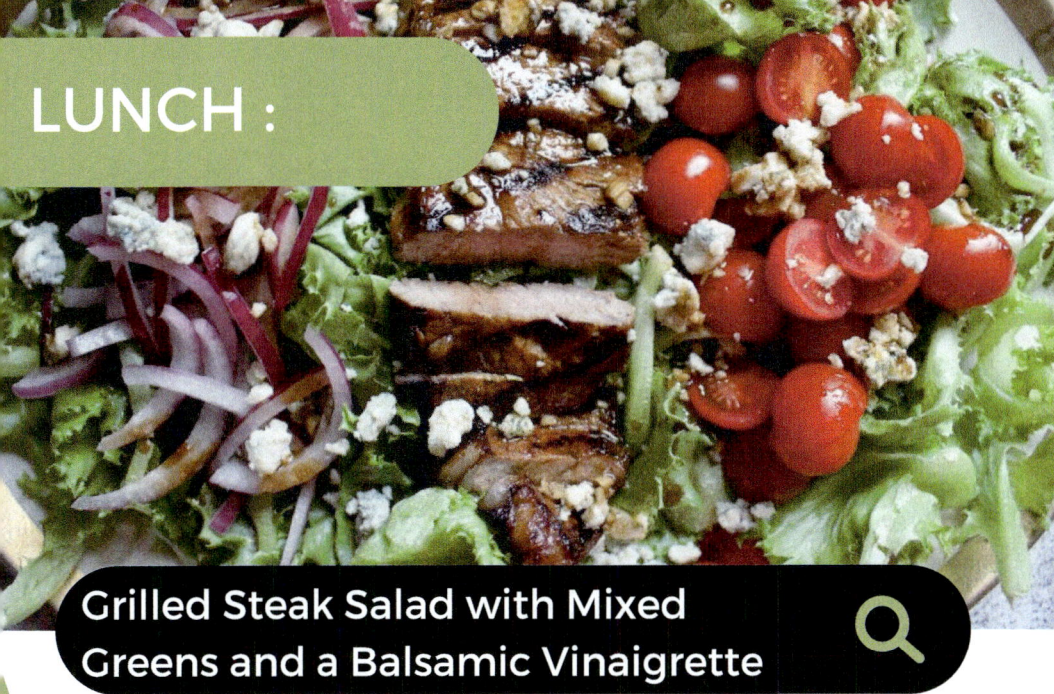

Grilled Steak Salad with Mixed Greens and a Balsamic Vinaigrette

INGREDIENTS

- 1 steak cut of your choice (about 6 oz)
- 2 cups mixed greens (like lettuce, arugula, spinach)
- 1/4 cup cherry tomatoes, halved
- 2 tablespoons olive oil
- 1 tablespoon balsamic vinegar
- Salt and pepper, to taste

PROCEDURE

- Season the steak with salt and pepper.
- Grill the steak over medium-high heat to your desired level of doneness, about 4-5 minutes per side for medium-rare.
- Let the steak rest for a few minutes, then slice it.
- In a bowl, toss the mixed greens and cherry tomatoes.
- Whisk together olive oil and balsamic vinegar for the dressing.
- Drizzle the dressing over the salad.
- Top the salad with the sliced grilled steak.
- Serve immediately for a fresh and hearty lunch.

DINNER :

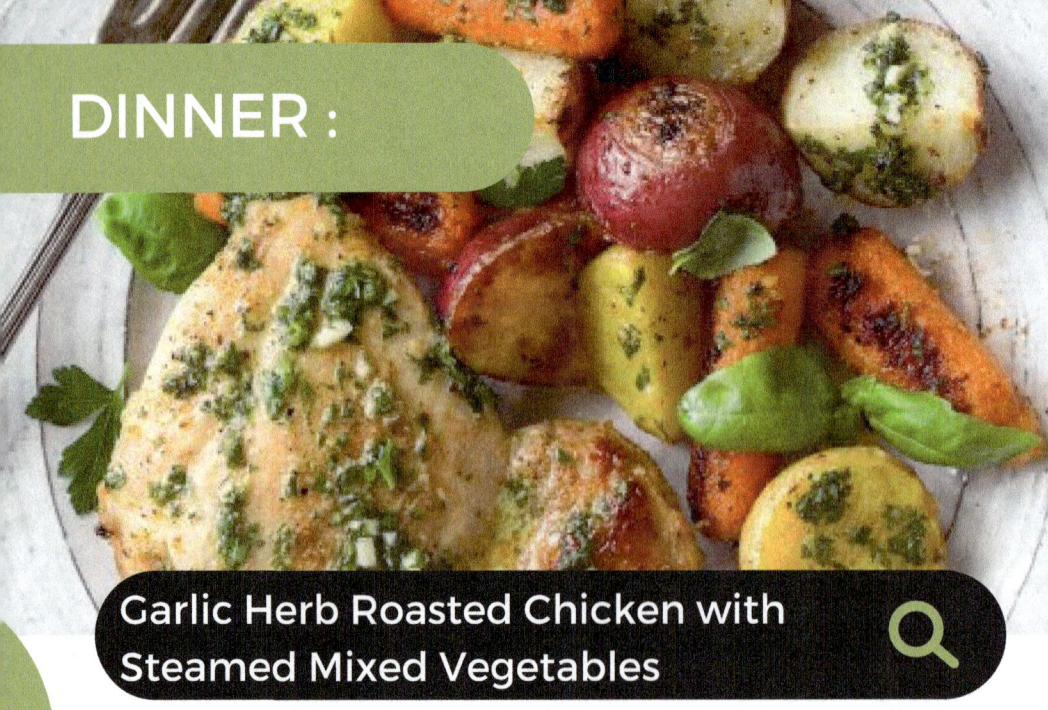

Garlic Herb Roasted Chicken with Steamed Mixed Vegetables

INGREDIENTS

- 1 small chicken breast
- 1 garlic clove, minced
- 1/2 teaspoon dried herbs (like thyme or rosemary)
- 1 tablespoon olive oil
- 1 cup mixed vegetables (broccoli, carrots, cauliflower)
- Salt and pepper, to taste

PROCEDURE

- Preheat the oven to 375°F (190°C).
- Rub the chicken breast with olive oil, minced garlic, dried herbs, salt, and pepper.
- Place the chicken in a baking dish and roast for 25-30 minutes, or until fully cooked.
- While the chicken is roasting, steam the mixed vegetables until tender, about 5-7 minutes.
- Season the vegetables with a little salt and pepper.
- Serve the garlic herb roasted chicken with the steamed mixed vegetables.

PALEO DIET

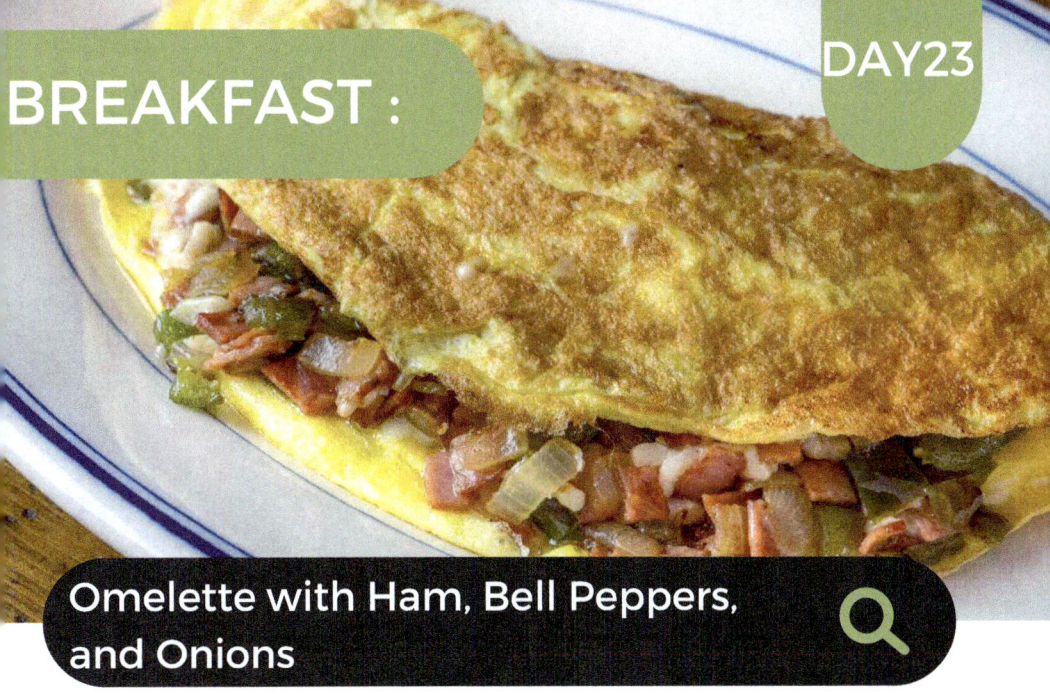

BREAKFAST :

DAY 23

Omelette with Ham, Bell Peppers, and Onions

INGREDIENTS

- 2 large eggs
- 1/4 cup ham, diced (ensure it's Paleo-friendly)
- 1/4 bell pepper, diced
- 1/4 onion, diced
- 1 tablespoon olive oil
- Salt and pepper, to taste

PROCEDURE

- Beat the eggs in a bowl and season with salt and pepper.
- Heat the olive oil in a skillet over medium heat.
- Sauté the bell pepper and onion until soft, about 3-4 minutes.
- Add the diced ham and cook for another minute.
- Pour the beaten eggs over the ham and vegetables.
- Cook without stirring for a few minutes until the bottom sets.
- Carefully fold the omelette in half and cook for another minute.
- Serve the omelette hot.

PALEO DIET

LUNCH :

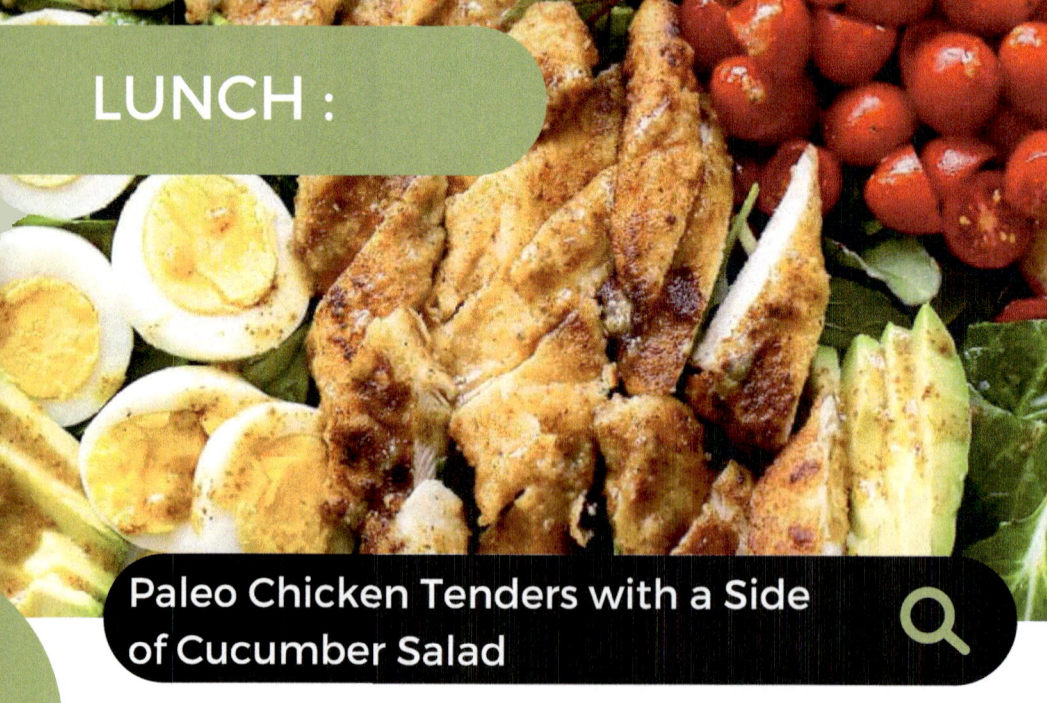

Paleo Chicken Tenders with a Side of Cucumber Salad

INGREDIENTS

- 1/2 lb chicken breast, cut into strips
- 1/4 cup almond flour
- 1 egg, beaten
- Salt and pepper, to taste
- 1 tablespoon olive oil for cooking

Ingredients for Cucumber Salad:
- 1 cucumber, sliced
- 2 tablespoons olive oil
- 1 tablespoon apple cider vinegar
- Salt and pepper, to taste

PROCEDURE

- Season the chicken strips with salt and pepper, then dip them in the beaten egg and coat with almond flour.
- Heat olive oil in a skillet and cook the chicken tenders over medium heat until golden and cooked through, about 3-4 minutes per side.
- In a bowl, mix together the sliced cucumber, olive oil, apple cider vinegar, salt, and pepper.
- Serve the chicken tenders with the cucumber salad on the side.

PALEO DIET

DINNER :

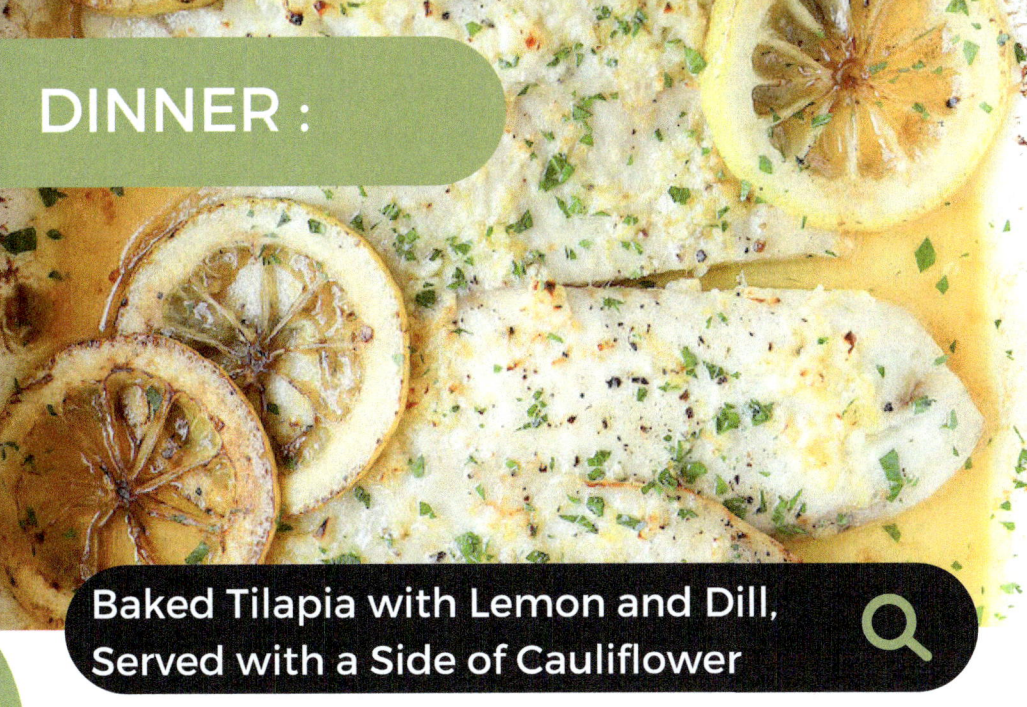

Baked Tilapia with Lemon and Dill, Served with a Side of Cauliflower

INGREDIENTS

- 1 tilapia fillet (about 6 oz)
- 1/2 lemon, juiced and zested
- 1 teaspoon fresh dill, chopped
- Salt and pepper, to taste

Ingredients for Cauliflower Mash:
- 1/2 head of cauliflower, cut into florets
- 1 tablespoon olive oil
- Salt and pepper, to taste

PROCEDURE

- Preheat the oven to 375°F (190°C).
- Place the tilapia on a baking sheet. Season with lemon juice, lemon zest, dill, salt, and pepper.
- Bake for 12-15 minutes, or until the fish flakes easily with a fork.
- Meanwhile, steam the cauliflower florets until tender, about 7-10 minutes.
- Blend the steamed cauliflower with olive oil, salt, and pepper until smooth to make cauliflower mash.
- Serve the baked tilapia with the cauliflower mash on the side.

PALEO DIET

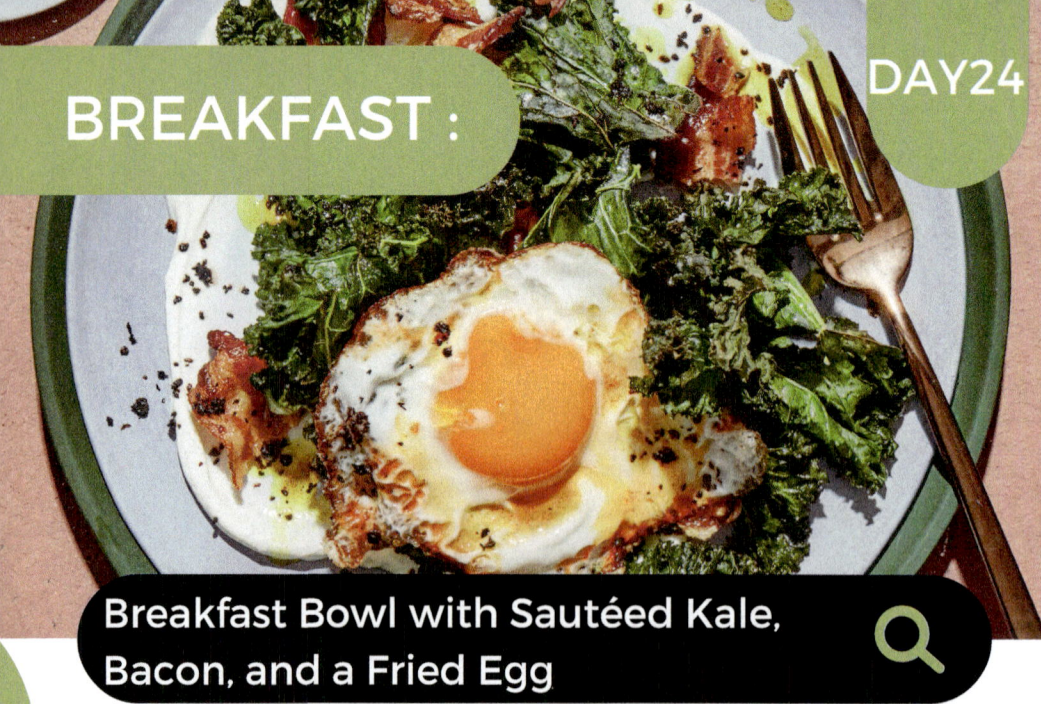

BREAKFAST:

DAY 24

Breakfast Bowl with Sautéed Kale, Bacon, and a Fried Egg

INGREDIENTS

- 1 cup kale, chopped
- 2 slices of bacon
- 1 large egg
- 1 tablespoon olive oil
- Salt and pepper, to taste

PROCEDURE

- Cook the bacon in a skillet over medium heat until crispy. Remove and set aside on a paper towel. Chop or crumble once cooled.
- In the same skillet, add the kale and sauté in the bacon fat until wilted, about 2-3 minutes. Season with salt and pepper.
- Remove the kale and set aside.
- Add a little olive oil to the skillet and fry the egg to your liking.
- Assemble the breakfast bowl with sautéed kale, crumbled bacon, and the fried egg on top.
- Serve hot for a hearty start to your day.

PALEO DIET

LUNCH :

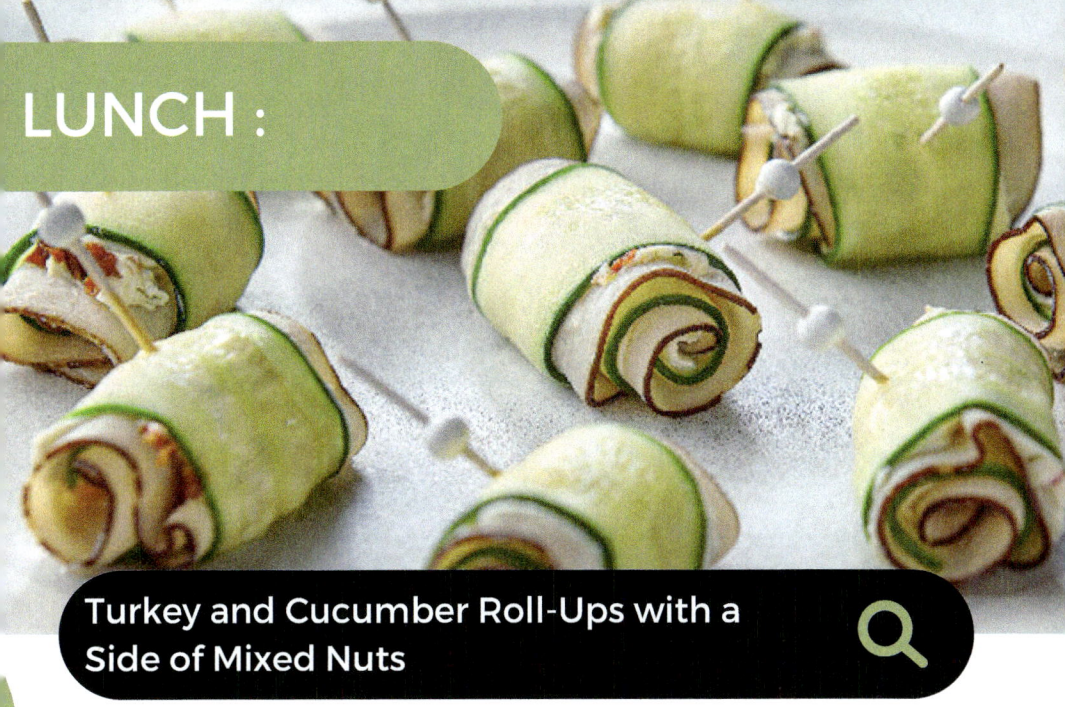

Turkey and Cucumber Roll-Ups with a Side of Mixed Nuts

INGREDIENTS

- 4-5 slices of turkey breast (ensure it's Paleo-friendly)
- 1/2 cucumber, thinly sliced lengthwise
- Mixed nuts (almonds, walnuts, cashews) - a small handful

PROCEDURE

- Lay out the turkey slices.
- Place a few cucumber slices on each turkey slice.
- Roll the turkey slices tightly around the cucumber.
- Serve with a side of mixed nuts.

PALEO DIET

DINNER :

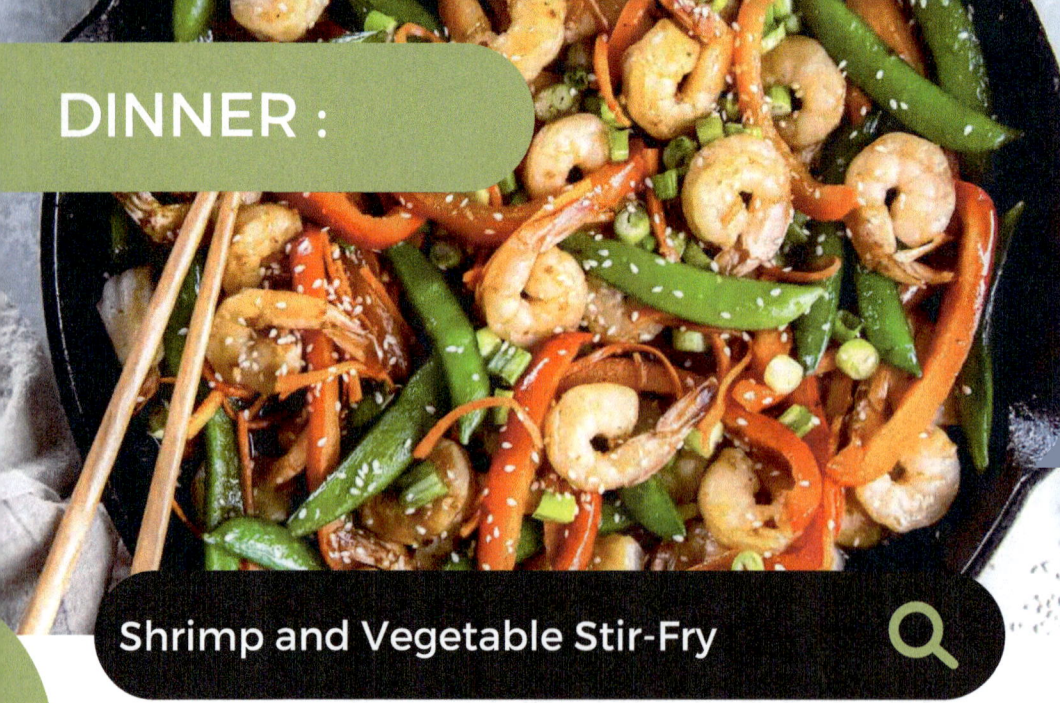

Shrimp and Vegetable Stir-Fry

INGREDIENTS

- 5-6 large shrimp, peeled and deveined
- 1 cup mixed vegetables (such as bell peppers, broccoli, and carrots), chopped
- 1 tablespoon coconut oil
- 1 garlic clove, minced
- 1 tablespoon soy sauce or coconut aminos
- Salt and pepper, to taste

PROCEDURE

- Heat coconut oil in a wok or large skillet over medium-high heat.
- Add garlic and sauté for about 30 seconds.
- Add the chopped vegetables and stir-fry until they begin to soften, about 3-4 minutes.
- Add the shrimp and cook until they turn pink and are cooked through, about 2-3 minutes.
- Add soy sauce or coconut aminos, and season with salt and pepper. Stir well to combine all ingredients.
- Serve the shrimp and vegetable stir-fry hot.

PALEO DIET

BREAKFAST :

DAY 25

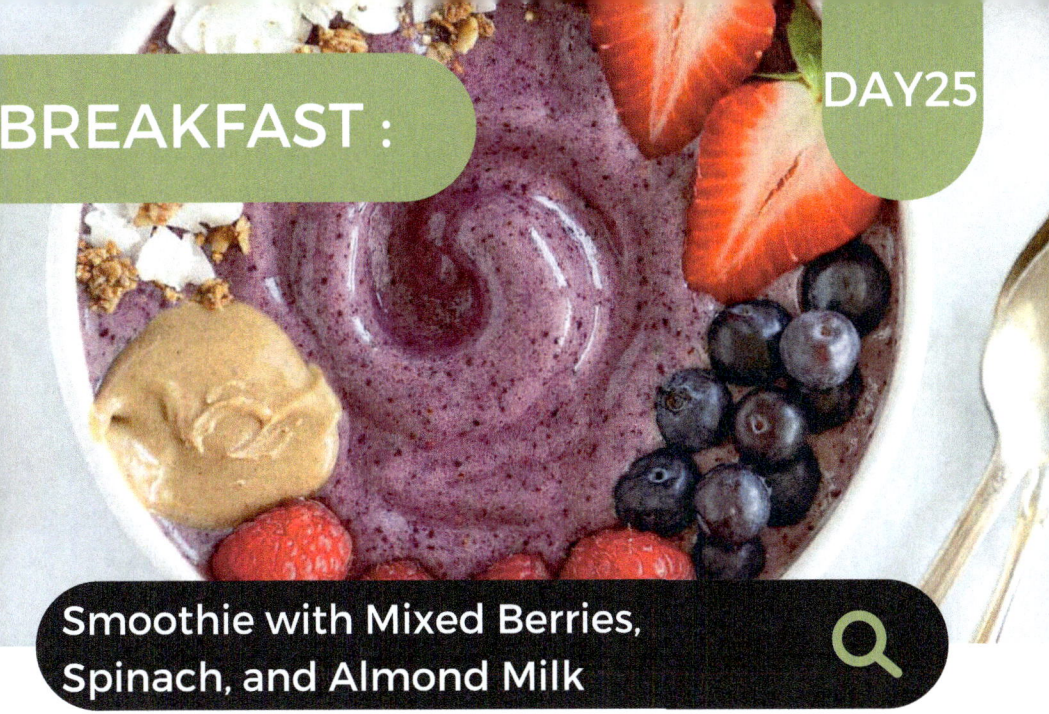

Smoothie with Mixed Berries, Spinach, and Almond Milk

INGREDIENTS

- 1/2 cup mixed berries (strawberries, blueberries, raspberries)
- 1 cup spinach
- 3/4 cup almond milk (unsweetened)
- Ice cubes (optional)

PROCEDURE

- Combine the mixed berries, spinach, and almond milk in a blender.
- Add ice cubes if desired for a colder smoothie.
- Blend until smooth and creamy.
- Serve immediately in a tall glass for a refreshing and nutritious start to your day.

PALEO DIET

LUNCH :

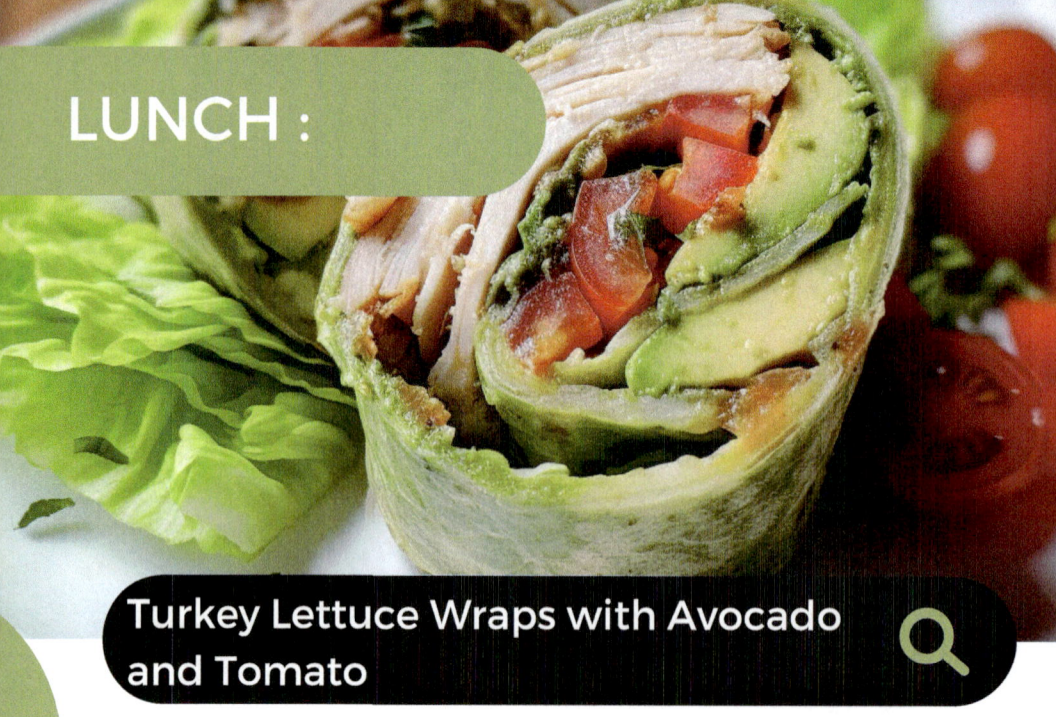

Turkey Lettuce Wraps with Avocado and Tomato

INGREDIENTS

- 4-5 slices of turkey breast (ensure it's Paleo-friendly)
- 1 avocado, sliced
- 1 tomato, sliced
- Large lettuce leaves (such as Romaine or Iceberg)
- Salt and pepper, to taste

PROCEDURE

- Lay out the lettuce leaves.
- Place a slice or two of turkey on each lettuce leaf.
- Add slices of avocado and tomato on top of the turkey.
- Season with salt and pepper.
- Roll up the lettuce leaves to form wraps.
- Serve immediately for a light and satisfying lunch.

DINNER :

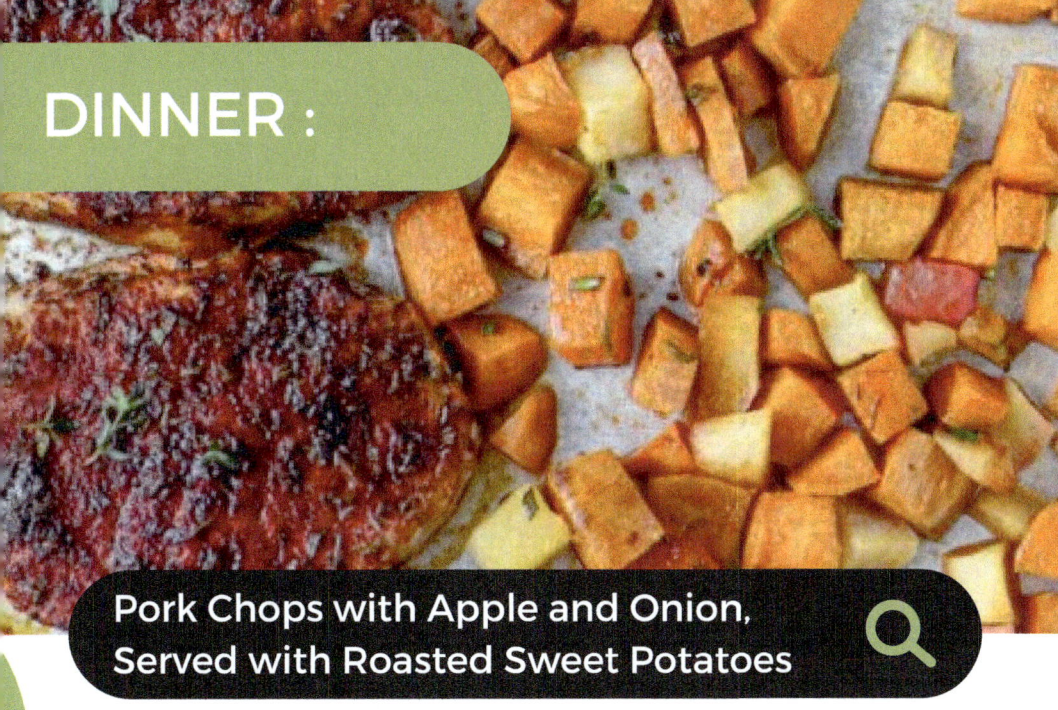

Pork Chops with Apple and Onion, Served with Roasted Sweet Potatoes

INGREDIENTS

- 2 pork chops
- 1 apple, sliced
- 1/2 onion, sliced
- 1 tablespoon olive oil
- Salt and pepper, to taste

Ingredients for Roasted Sweet Potatoes:
- 1 large sweet potato, peeled and cubed
- 1 tablespoon olive oil
- Salt and pepper, to taste

PROCEDURE

- Preheat the oven to 400°F (200°C).
- Season the pork chops with salt and pepper.
- Heat olive oil in a skillet over medium-high heat. Add the pork chops and cook until browned on both sides.
- Add the sliced apple and onion to the skillet with the pork chops.
- Transfer the skillet to the oven and roast for about 10-15 minutes, until the pork chops are cooked through.
- For the sweet potatoes, toss them with olive oil, salt, and pepper, and spread on a baking sheet.
- Roast in the oven for about 20-25 minutes, until tender and lightly caramelized.
- Serve the pork chops with the apple and onion alongside the roasted sweet potatoes.

PALEO DIET

BREAKFAST :

DAY26

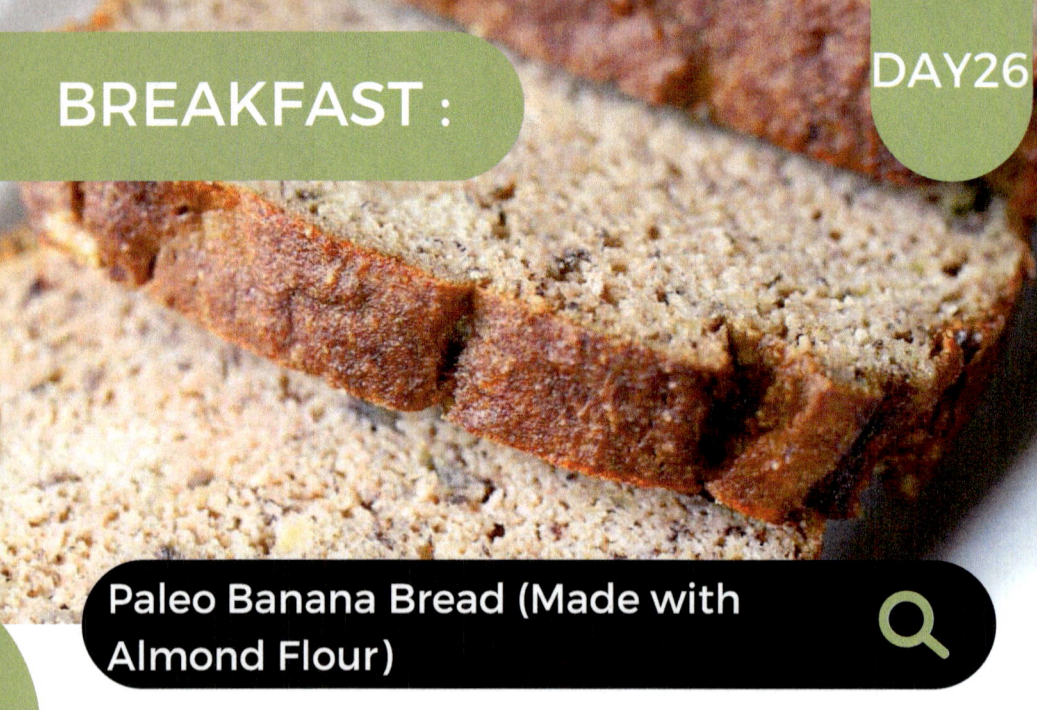

Paleo Banana Bread (Made with Almond Flour)

INGREDIENTS

- 1 ripe banana, mashed
- 2 cups almond flour
- 3 large eggs
- 1/4 cup honey or maple syrup
- 1/4 cup coconut oil, melted
- 1 teaspoon baking powder
- 1/2 teaspoon cinnamon
- Pinch of salt

PROCEDURE

- Preheat the oven to 350°F (175°C) and line a loaf pan with parchment paper.
- In a bowl, mix together the mashed banana, eggs, honey or maple syrup, and melted coconut oil.
- Add the almond flour, baking powder, cinnamon, and a pinch of salt to the wet ingredients. Stir until well combined.
- Pour the batter into the prepared loaf pan.
- Bake for about 30-35 minutes, or until a toothpick inserted into the center comes out clean.
- Let the banana bread cool before slicing and serving.

PALEO DIET

LUNCH :

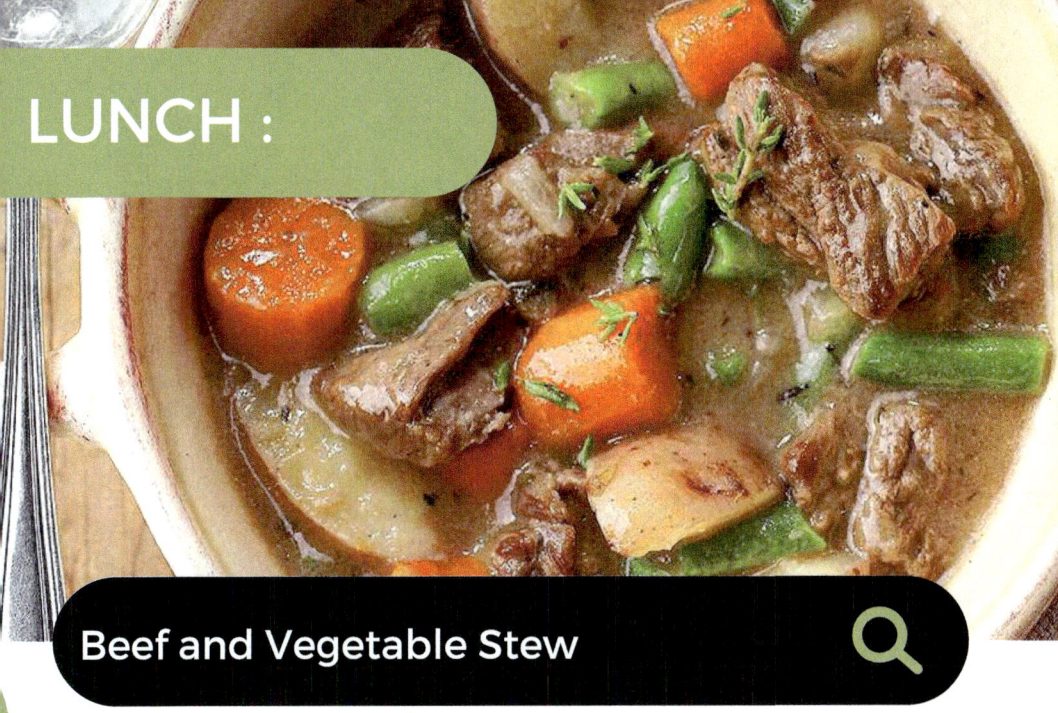

Beef and Vegetable Stew

INGREDIENTS

- 1/2 lb beef stew meat, cut into cubes
- 2 cups beef broth (Paleo-friendly)
- 1 cup mixed vegetables (carrots, celery, onions)
- 1 garlic clove, minced
- 1 tablespoon tomato paste (check for no added sugar)
- 1 tablespoon olive oil
- Salt and pepper, to taste
- Herbs (like thyme or rosemary), to taste

PROCEDURE

- Heat the olive oil in a pot over medium-high heat. Brown the beef cubes on all sides. Remove and set aside.
- In the same pot, add the garlic and vegetables. Cook until softened.
- Return the beef to the pot. Add the beef broth, tomato paste, herbs, salt, and pepper.
- Bring to a boil, then reduce heat and simmer for about 1-1.5 hours, until the beef is tender.
- Adjust seasoning as needed and serve hot.

DINNER :

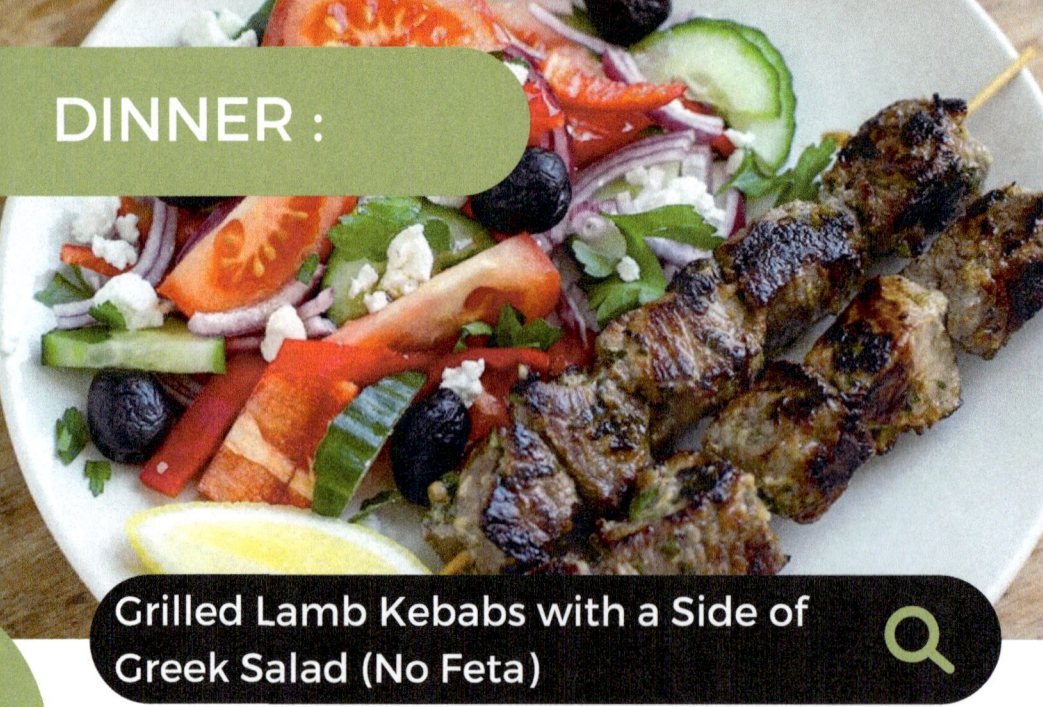

Grilled Lamb Kebabs with a Side of Greek Salad (No Feta)

INGREDIENTS

- 1/2 lb lamb, cut into cubes
- 1 tablespoon olive oil
- 1 teaspoon dried oregano
- Salt and pepper, to taste

Ingredients for Greek Salad:
- 1 cucumber, diced
- 1 tomato, diced
- 1/4 red onion, thinly sliced
- 1/4 cup olives, pitted
- 2 tablespoons olive oil
- 1 tablespoon red wine vinegar
- Salt and pepper, to taste

PROCEDURE

- Preheat the grill to medium-high heat.
- Toss the lamb cubes with olive oil, oregano, salt, and pepper.
- Thread the lamb onto skewers and grill for about 10-12 minutes, turning occasionally, until cooked to your liking.
- For the salad, combine cucumber, tomato, red onion, and olives in a bowl.
- Dress the salad with olive oil, red wine vinegar, salt, and pepper.
- Serve the grilled lamb kebabs with the Greek salad on the side.

PALEO DIET

BREAKFAST :

DAY 27

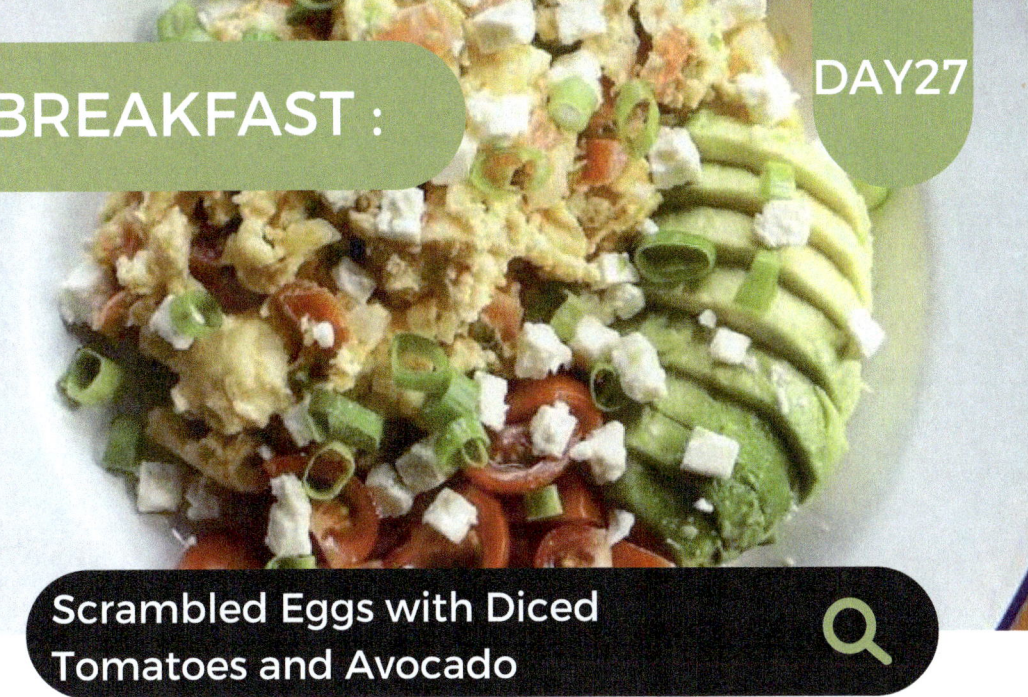

Scrambled Eggs with Diced Tomatoes and Avocado

INGREDIENTS

- 2 large eggs
- 1 small tomato, diced
- 1/2 ripe avocado, diced
- 1 tablespoon olive oil
- Salt and pepper, to taste

PROCEDURE

- Beat the eggs in a bowl and season with salt and pepper.
- Heat the olive oil in a skillet over medium heat.
- Add the diced tomato to the skillet and cook for about 1-2 minutes.
- Pour the beaten eggs over the tomatoes.
- Scramble the eggs until they are just set.
- Remove from heat and gently fold in the diced avocado.
- Serve the scrambled eggs warm.

LUNCH :

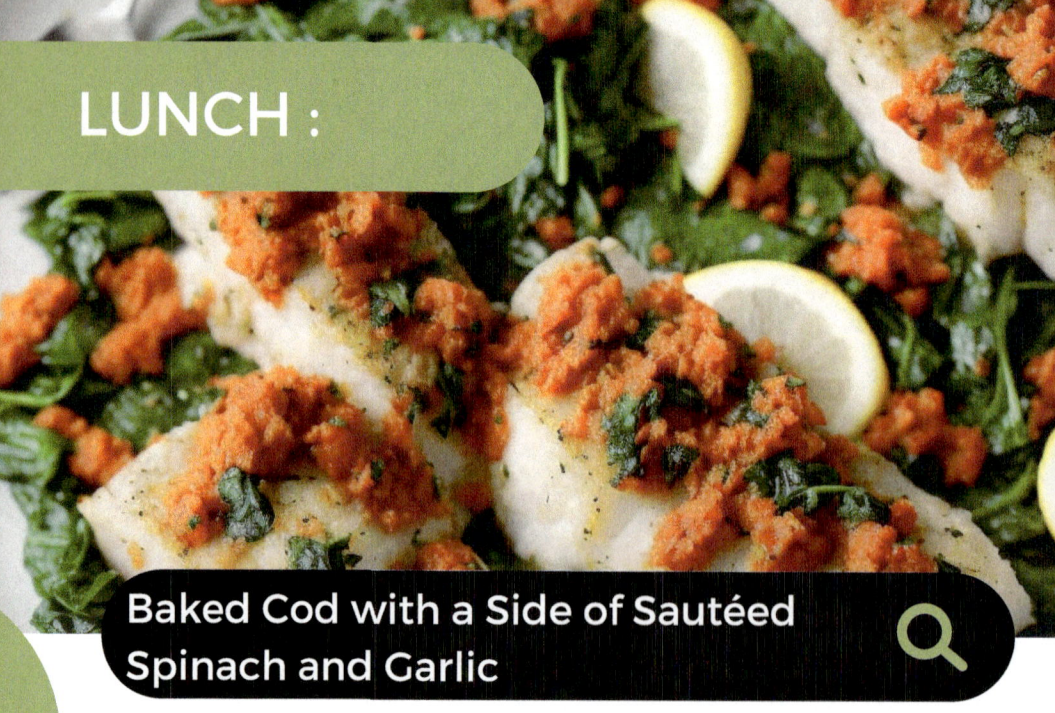

Baked Cod with a Side of Sautéed Spinach and Garlic

INGREDIENTS

- 1 cod fillet (about 6 oz)
- 1 tablespoon olive oil
- 1/2 lemon, juiced
- Salt and pepper, to taste

Ingredients for Sautéed Spinach:
- 2 cups spinach
- 1 garlic clove, minced
- 1 tablespoon olive oil
- Salt and pepper, to taste

PROCEDURE

- Preheat the oven to 375°F (190°C).
- Place the cod fillet on a baking sheet and drizzle with olive oil and lemon juice. Season with salt and pepper.
- Bake for 12-15 minutes, or until the fish flakes easily with a fork.
- For the spinach, heat olive oil in a skillet over medium heat.
- Add minced garlic and sauté for 30 seconds.
- Add the spinach and cook until wilted, about 2-3 minutes. Season with salt and pepper.
- Serve the baked cod with the sautéed spinach on the side.

PALEO DIET

DINNER :

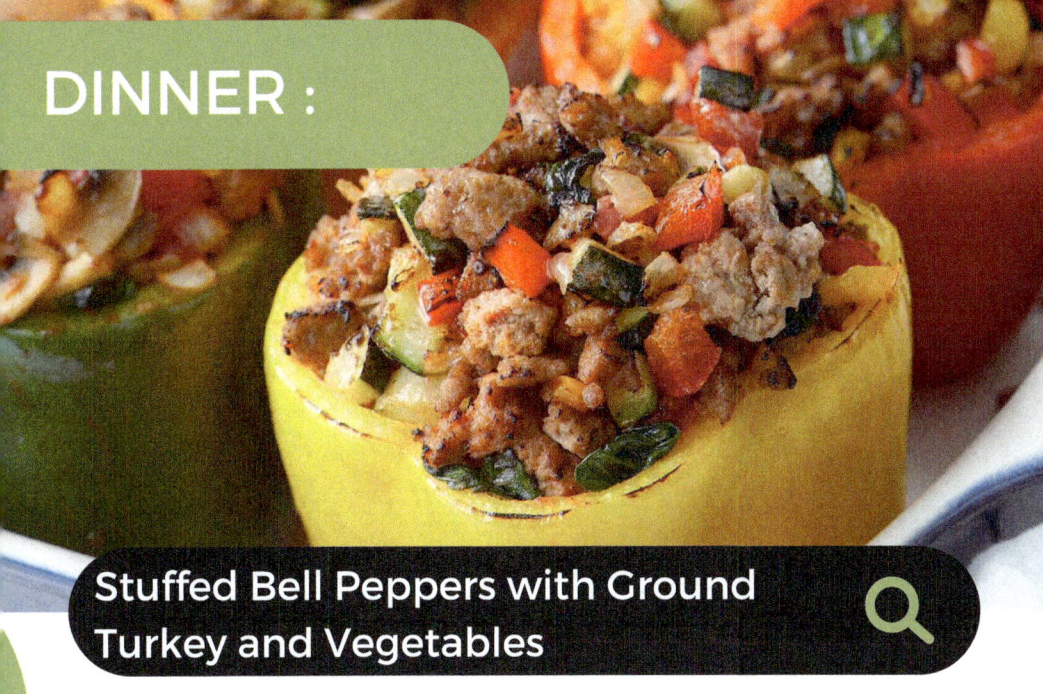

Stuffed Bell Peppers with Ground Turkey and Vegetables

INGREDIENTS

- 2 bell peppers, halved and seeds removed
- 1/2 lb ground turkey
- 1/2 onion, diced
- 1/2 cup mushrooms, chopped
- 1 garlic clove, minced
- 1 tablespoon olive oil
- Salt and pepper, to taste
- 1/2 cup Paleo-friendly tomato sauce

PROCEDURE

- Preheat the oven to 375°F (190°C).
- In a skillet, heat olive oil over medium heat. Add the ground turkey, onion, mushrooms, and garlic. Cook until the turkey is browned.
- Stir in the tomato sauce and season with salt and pepper.
- Spoon the turkey and vegetable mixture into the bell pepper halves.
- Place the stuffed peppers in a baking dish and bake for 25-30 minutes, until the peppers are tender.
- Serve the stuffed bell peppers warm.

PALEO DIET

BREAKFAST :

DAY28

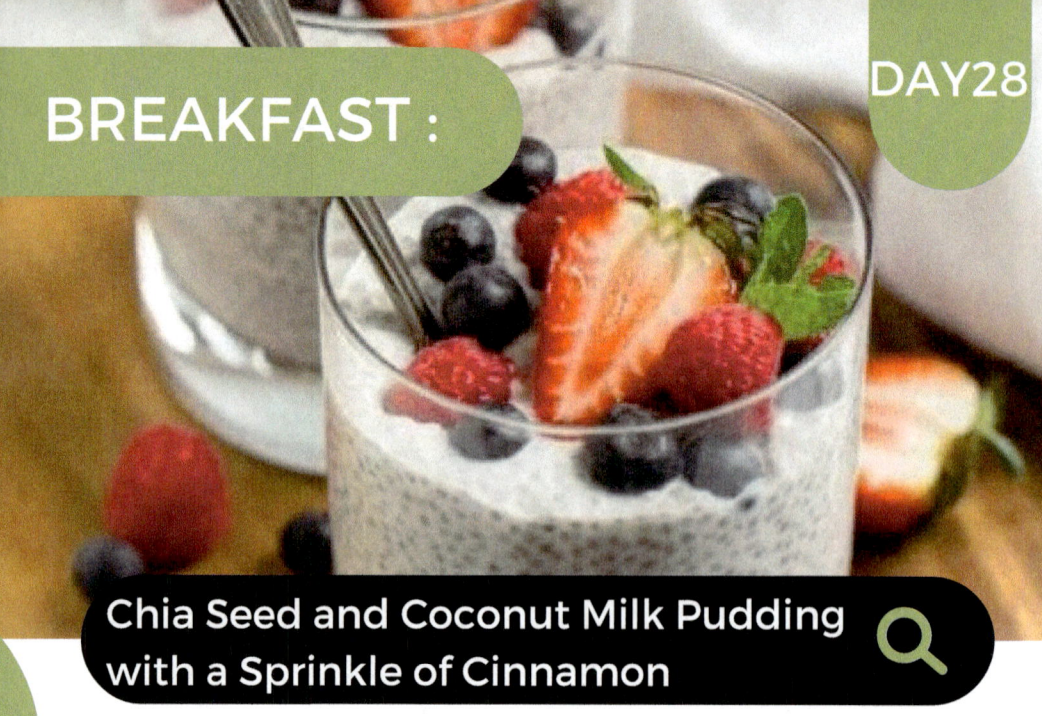

Chia Seed and Coconut Milk Pudding with a Sprinkle of Cinnamon

INGREDIENTS

- 3 tablespoons chia seeds
- 3/4 cup coconut milk (unsweetened)
- 1/2 teaspoon vanilla extract (optional)
- 1 tablespoon honey or maple syrup (optional)
- A sprinkle of cinnamon

PROCEDURE

- In a bowl, mix the chia seeds with coconut milk, vanilla extract (if using), and honey or maple syrup (if using).
- Stir well to combine and let sit for 5 minutes, then stir again to prevent clumping.
- Cover and refrigerate for at least 2 hours, preferably overnight, until it achieves a pudding-like consistency.
- Before serving, sprinkle with cinnamon for added flavor.

PALEO DIET

LUNCH :

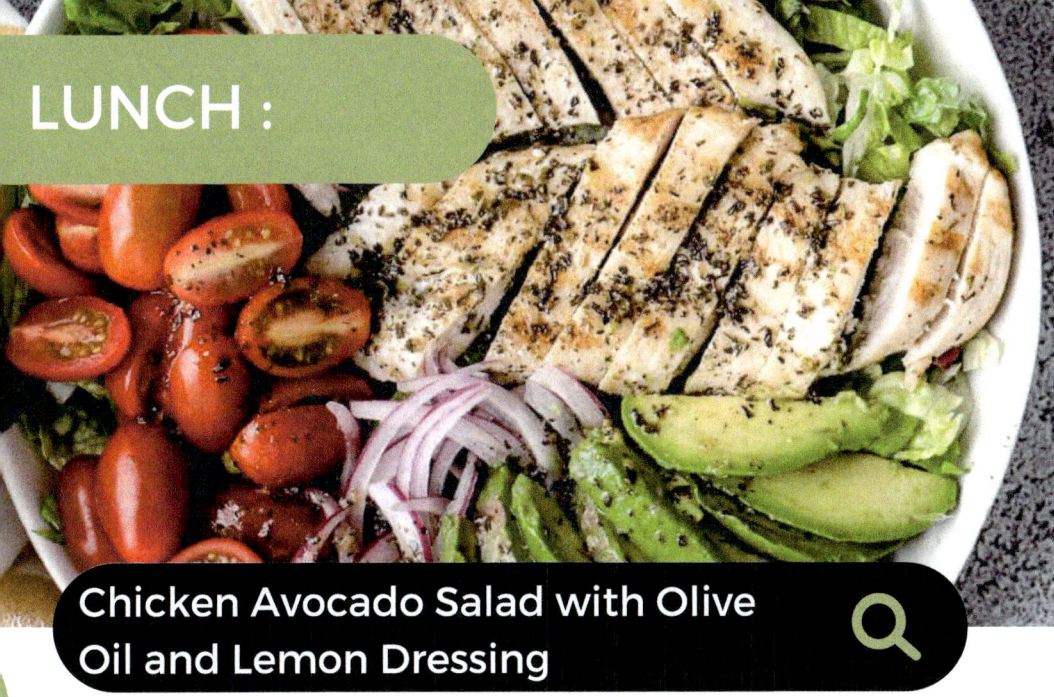

Chicken Avocado Salad with Olive Oil and Lemon Dressing

INGREDIENTS

- 1 small chicken breast, grilled and sliced
- 1 avocado, diced
- 2 cups mixed greens (like lettuce, arugula, spinach)
- 2 tablespoons olive oil
- 1 tablespoon lemon juice
- Salt and pepper, to taste

PROCEDURE

- In a large bowl, place the mixed greens, sliced grilled chicken, and diced avocado.
- In a small bowl, whisk together olive oil, lemon juice, salt, and pepper to make a dressing.
- Drizzle the dressing over the salad.
- Toss gently to combine.
- Serve immediately for a refreshing and satisfying lunch.

DINNER :

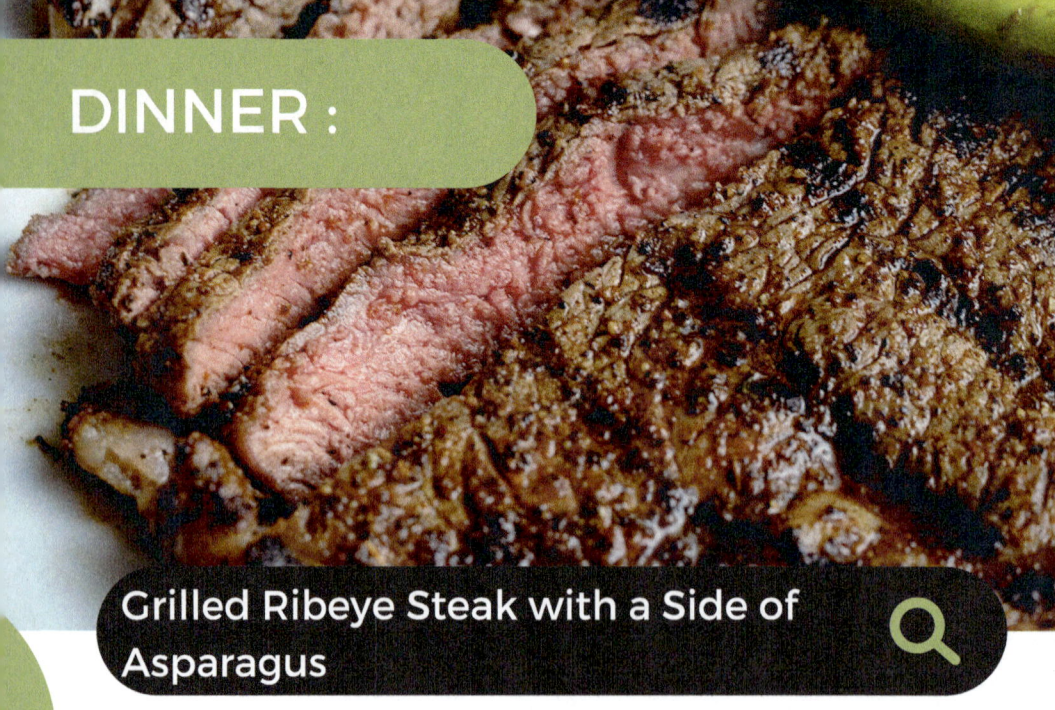

Grilled Ribeye Steak with a Side of Asparagus

INGREDIENTS

- 1 ribeye steak (about 6-8 oz)
- 1 cup asparagus spears, ends trimmed
- 1 tablespoon olive oil
- Salt and pepper, to taste

PROCEDURE

- Season the ribeye steak with salt and pepper.
- Preheat your grill to medium-high heat.
- Grill the steak to your preferred level of doneness, about 4-5 minutes per side for medium-rare.
- In the meantime, toss the asparagus with olive oil and season with salt and pepper.
- Grill the asparagus alongside the steak until tender and slightly charred, about 2-3 minutes per side.
- Let the steak rest for a few minutes before slicing.
- Serve the grilled ribeye steak with the grilled asparagus.

PALEO DIET

After completing Week 4, it's important to reflect on how your body has responded to the dietary changes. Use the following scale to rate your experiences in various aspects of your health and well-being. Rate each category from 1 to 10 (where 1 is 'no improvement' and 10 is 'significant improvement').

1. Digestive Comfort
- Question: How would you rate the overall comfort of your digestive system this week?
- Rating (1-10): _____

2. Energy Levels
- Question: How do you feel about your energy levels after following the meal plan for a week?
- Rating (1-10): _____

3. Sleep Quality
- Question: Have you noticed any changes in the quality of your sleep?
- Rating (1-10): _____

4. Mood and Mental Clarity
- Question: How has your mood and mental clarity been affected by the dietary changes?
- Rating (1-10): _____

5. Physical Comfort and Pain Levels
- Question: If you previously experienced any physical discomfort or pain, have you noticed any changes in its intensity or frequency?
- Rating (1-10): _____

6. Skin Health
- Question: Have there been any noticeable changes in your skin health/appearance?
- Rating (1-10): _____

7. Cravings and Appetite Control
- Question: How would you rate your control over cravings and appetite this week?
- Rating (1-10): _____

8. Overall Well-being
- Question: Considering all factors, how would you rate your overall well-being after Week 1?
- Rating (1-10): _____

WEEK 1

DIGESTIVE COMFORT	1	2	3	4	5	6	7	8	9	10
ENERGY LEVELS	1	2	3	4	5	6	7	8	9	10
SLEEP QUALITY	1	2	3	4	5	6	7	8	9	10
MOOD & MENTAL CLARITY	1	2	3	4	5	6	7	8	9	10
PHYSICAL COMFORT	1	2	3	4	5	6	7	8	9	10
SKIN HEALTH	1	2	3	4	5	6	7	8	9	10
CRAVINGS CONTROL	1	2	3	4	5	6	7	8	9	10
OVERALL WELL-BEING	1	2	3	4	5	6	7	8	9	10

notes

PALEO DIET

FOR SPECIAL *notes*

SNACKS

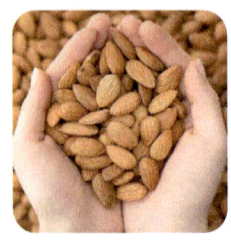

DAY 1

A Handful of Almonds

Simply measure out a small handful of raw or roasted almonds (about 1/4 cup) to enjoy as a snack. No preparation is needed.

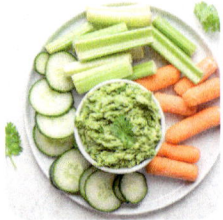

DAY 2

Sliced Cucumber and Carrots with Guacamole

Ingredients:
- 1/2 cucumber, sliced
- 1 carrot, peeled and sliced
- 1/4 ripe avocado
- 1 teaspoon lime juice
- Salt and pepper, to taste

Instructions:
- Mash the avocado in a small bowl.
- Add lime juice, salt, and pepper to the mashed avocado to make a simple guacamole.
- Serve the guacamole with sliced cucumber and carrot sticks.

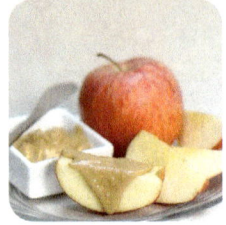

DAY 2

Apple Slices with Almond Butter

Simply slice one apple and serve with a tablespoon of almond butter for dipping.

PALEO DIET

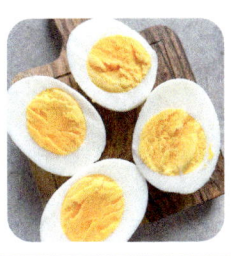

DAY 4

Hard-Boiled Eggs

Boil 1-2 eggs by placing them in a pot of water, bringing it to a boil, and then letting them cook for 9-12 minutes for hard-boiled eggs. Cool in ice water, peel, and enjoy as a snack.

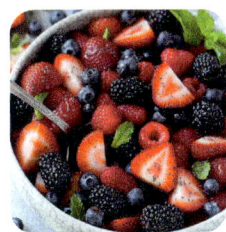

DAY 5

A Small Bowl of Mixed Berries

Combine a mix of berries such as strawberries, blueberries, raspberries, and blackberries in a small bowl. Enjoy fresh and chilled.

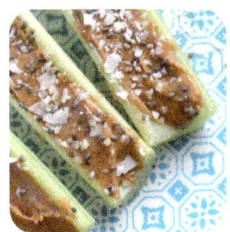

DAY 6

Celery Sticks with Almond Butter

- Simply wash and cut 2-3 celery stalks into sticks.
- Serve with a tablespoon of almond butter for dipping.

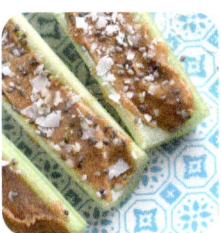

DAY 7

A Handful of Macadamia Nuts

Measure out a small handful of macadamia nuts (about 1/4 cup) to enjoy as a snack. No preparation is needed.

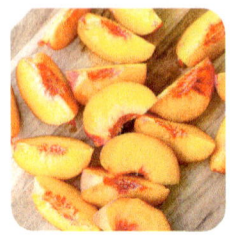

DAY 8

Fresh Peach Slices

Simply wash and slice one fresh peach. Enjoy the slices as a sweet and refreshing snack.

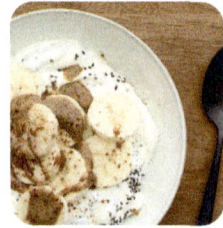

DAY 9

Banana with a Spoonful of Almond Butter

Peel a banana and serve with a tablespoon of almond butter for dipping.

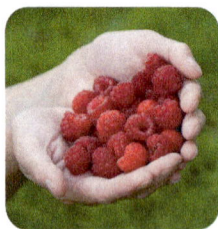

DAY 10

A Handful of Raspberries

Simply enjoy a small handful of fresh raspberries as a light and refreshing snack.

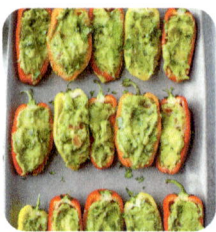

DAY 11

Sliced Bell Peppers with Guacamole

- 1/2 bell pepper, sliced
- 1/4 ripe avocado
- 1 teaspoon lime juice
- Salt and pepper, to taste

PALEO DIET

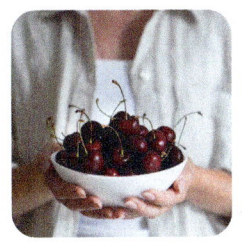

DAY 12

A Small Bowl of Cherries

Serve a small bowl of fresh cherries as a sweet and simple snack. Make sure to wash them before eating.

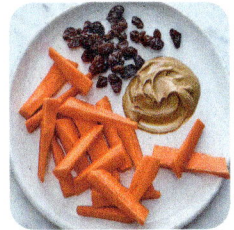

DAY 13

Carrot Sticks with Almond Butter

- Peel and cut 1-2 carrots into sticks.
- Serve with a tablespoon of almond butter for dipping.

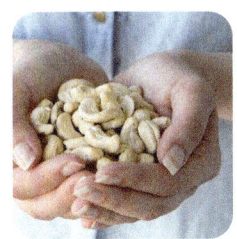

DAY 14

A Handful of Cashews

Enjoy a small handful of raw or roasted cashews as a simple and satisfying snack.

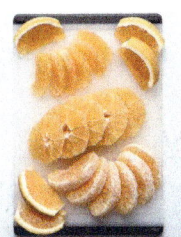

DAY 15 Orange Slices

Peel and section one orange, and enjoy the slices as a refreshing and sweet snack.

PALEO DIET

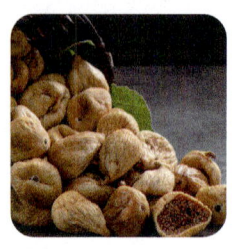

DAY 16

A Handful of Dried Figs

Enjoy a small handful of dried figs as a nutritious and sweet snack. Ensure they are unsweetened and without any added preservatives to stay within Paleo guidelines.

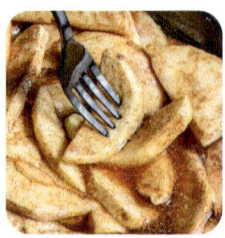

DAY 17

Sliced Apple with Cinnamon

Slice one apple and sprinkle with a dash of cinnamon for a simple and healthy snack.

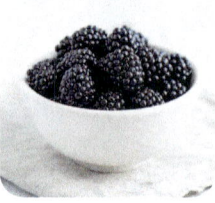

DAY 18

A Small Bowl of Blackberries

Serve a small bowl of fresh blackberries as a light and nutritious snack. Wash them thoroughly before eating.

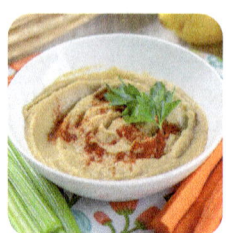

DAY 19 Celery Sticks with Tahini

- Wash and cut 2-3 celery stalks into sticks.
- Serve with a tablespoon of tahini (sesame seed paste) for dipping.

PALEO DIET

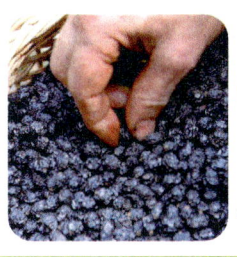

DAY 20

A Handful of Olives

Enjoy a small handful of olives as a savory and healthy snack. Choose a variety that suits your preference, such as Kalamata or green olives.

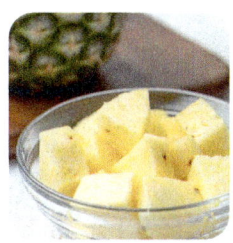

DAY 21

A Small Bowl of Pineapple Chunks

Cut a fresh pineapple into chunks and serve in a small bowl for a sweet and tropical snack.

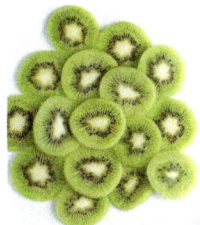

DAY 22

Sliced Kiwi

Peel and slice one or two kiwi fruits for a refreshing and vitamin-rich snack.

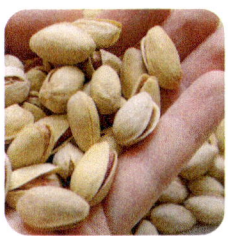

DAY 23 — A Handful of Pistachios

Enjoy a small handful of shelled pistachios as a healthy and satisfying snack.

PALEO DIET

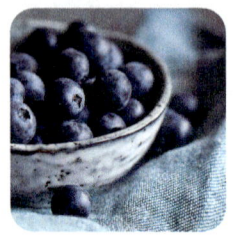

DAY 24

A Small Bowl of Blueberries

Serve a small bowl of fresh blueberries as a light and nutritious snack. Wash them thoroughly before eating.

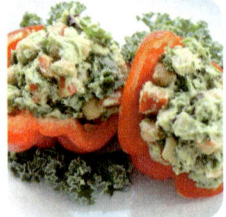

DAY 25

Sliced Bell Pepper with Guacamole

- 1 bell pepper, sliced
- 1/4 ripe avocado
- 1 teaspoon lime juice
- Salt and pepper, to taste

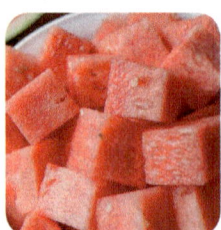

DAY 26

A Small Bowl of Melon Cubes

Cut a variety of melon (like cantaloupe, honeydew, or watermelon) into cubes and serve in a small bowl for a refreshing and hydrating snack.

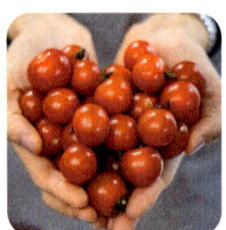

DAY 27

A Handful of Cherry Tomatoes

Enjoy a small handful of fresh cherry tomatoes as a light and flavorful snack. Wash them thoroughly before eating.

PALEO DIET

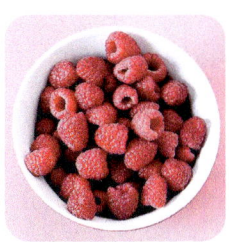

DAY 28

A Small Bowl of Raspberries

Serve a small bowl of fresh raspberries as a light and sweet snack. Wash them thoroughly before eating.

COMPLETION OF YOUR PALEO JOURNEY - A HEARTFELT THANK YOU

I want to express my deepest gratitude for your commitment and resilience throughout this Paleo journey. Remember, this isn't the end; it's a continuous path of exploration and fine-tuning. The insights and habits you've cultivated over the past four weeks are valuable tools that will empower you to maintain a nourishing and fulfilling lifestyle. Congratulations on this incredible accomplishment! As you move forward, keep reflecting on your progress with the Paleo Journey Progress Table.

PALEO JOURNEY PROGRESS TABLE

This table is designed to help you visually track and compare your experiences and health improvements over the four weeks of the diet. It will allow you to see the changes in various aspects of your health and well-being, helping you to understand the impact of the Paleo diet on your body and mind.

SECTION 4: WHAT NEXT

Congratulations on completing the 28-day Paleo meal plan! You've made significant strides in adopting a healthier lifestyle. But remember, this is just the beginning of a longer, more rewarding journey. Here's what you can do next to continue thriving on your Paleo path.

Reflect and Reassess:
- Evaluate Your Experience: Reflect on the last 28 days. Consider the changes in your health, your favorite meals, and how your body has responded to the diet. Did you discover any food sensitivities or particularly beneficial foods?
- Listen to Your Body: Continue to be attuned to how different foods affect you. This ongoing process will help you customize your Paleo diet to best suit your individual needs and health goals.

2. Continue Learning and Experimenting:
- Expand Your Recipe Collection: Variety is crucial in any sustainable diet. Websites like "Nom Nom Paleo" or "PaleOMG" offer a plethora of creative Paleo recipes. Try incorporating new recipes each week to keep your diet exciting and diverse.
- Educational Resources: To deepen your understanding of the Paleo lifestyle, consider resources like "The Paleo Solution" by Robb Wolf or "The Primal Blueprint" by Mark Sisson. Podcasts such as "The Paleo Solution Podcast" and "Revolution Health Radio" can also offer valuable insights and tips.

3. Set New Goals:
- Short-Term and Long-Term Goals: Based on your initial experience, set achievable goals. These could range from mastering specific Paleo recipes, to improving your fitness levels, to integrating more mindfulness practices into your daily routine.
- Track Progress: Tools like the Paleo Journey Progress Table or a journal are excellent for tracking your progress. Apps like "MyFitnessPal" can be adapted for Paleo tracking and can help monitor your dietary intake and physical activity.

WEEKS

	WEEK 1	WEEK 2	WEEK 3	WEEK 4
DIGESTIVE COMFORT				
ENERGY LEVELS				
SLEEP QUALITY				
MOOD & MENTAL CLARITY				
PHYSICAL COMFORT				
SKIN HEALTH				
CRAVINGS CONTROL				
OVERALL WELL-BEING				

notes

....
....
....
....
....

PALEO DIET

4. Build a Supportive Community:
   - Connect with Others: Online forums such as Reddit's r/Paleo community or The Paleo Diet®'s social media pages are great places to connect with fellow Paleo enthusiasts. Sharing experiences, challenges, and successes can provide motivation and support.
   - Involve Friends and Family: Encourage your loved ones to join you in your Paleo journey. Cooking Paleo meals together or sharing recipes can foster a supportive environment and make your lifestyle more enjoyable.
   -

5. Integrate Fitness and Lifestyle Changes:
   - Incorporate Regular Exercise: Exercise is a cornerstone of the Paleo lifestyle. Explore activities that you enjoy, be it weightlifting, yoga, hiking, or high-intensity interval training (HIIT). Resources like "Fitness Blender" offer a variety of free workout videos suitable for different fitness levels.
   - Mindfulness and Stress Management: Incorporate practices like meditation, yoga, or spending time in nature. Apps like "Headspace" or "Calm" offer guided meditation sessions that can help reduce stress and improve overall well-being.
   -

6. Plan for Challenges and Setbacks:
   - Develop Strategies: Anticipate potential challenges such as dining out or holiday meals. Websites like "The Paleo Mom" provide useful tips for navigating social situations while sticking to your diet.
   - Be Kind to Yourself: Understand that setbacks are a natural part of any lifestyle change. Be patient and view challenges as opportunities for growth. Remember, it's about progress, not perfection.

Your Paleo journey is a lifelong path of discovery, growth, and adjustment. Embrace it as an opportunity to continuously improve your health, learn more about your body, and enjoy a fulfilling lifestyle. Use the resources and strategies outlined here to stay informed, inspired, and on track. Here's to your health and happiness on the Paleo path!

BNW
PUBLISH

Join us on your favourite platform, Scan the QR code on your phone or tablet

THANK YOU

please review

on amazon

Printed in Great Britain
by Amazon

47407143R20076